GIVE YOUR DOG A BONE

The Practical Commonsense

Way to Feed Dogs

For a Long Healthy Life

Dr. Ian Billinghurst

PUBLISHED BY
IAN BILLINGHURST
"GIVE YOUR DOG A BONE"
P.O. BOX 703 LITHGOW
N.S.W. AUSTRALIA 2790

D0912706

First published in Australia 1993
by Ian Billinghurst
Fifth printing

Address all enquiries to
"Give Your Dog a Bone"
P.O. Box 703 Lithgow N.S.W.
Australia 2790

This book is an Australian product
Design and Typesetting by Ian Billinghurst
Illustrations by Jacqueline Castell
Photography by Elizabeth Castell
Edited by Elizabeth Shearman
Printed in Australia by Bridge Printery,
29-35 Dunning Avenue, Rosebery, NSW 2018
ISBN 0 646 16028 1

Contents

Note to Readers

The following information is supplied on the understanding that it is not designed to take the place of your Veterinarian. It's aim is to supplement your Veterinarian's advice and guidance. Diagnosis of a medical or surgical condition in your dog can only be carried out by a Veterinary Surgeon. The writer of this book cannot be responsible for decisions any reader may make with regard to feeding or treating their dog[s]. Any application of the recommendations set forth in the following pages is at the reader's discretion and sole risk. It is strongly advised that the reader at all times seeks out the best Veterinary resources available, in order that informed decisions on the care of dogs is obtained at all times.

- Acknowledgements -

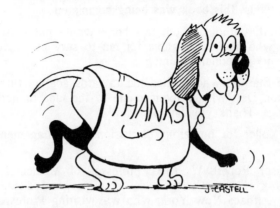

Thanks are due to many people, and many dogs, who have directly and indirectly contributed to this book. At the very least, they include the following.

The dogs that have shared their lives with me, starting with Candy my first-ever dog. She set me on the right track as regards the food requirements of healthy dogs. After Candy came Trixie, Sandy, Elizabeth, Dusty, Panda, Killa, Thunda, Molly, George, Teagan, Boris, Jaffa, Foxie, Scaredy Cat, Ruby, Dusty, Ben, Mouse, Bonnie, Yootha, Joyce, Poodle and Rupert.

The many other dogs who have stayed and walked and run and eaten with us for part of their lives, before moving on to their new owners. Every one of those dogs has made it's own unique contribution to our nutritional knowledge.

My client's dogs and my clients. They too have taught me much. From becoming acquainted with the feeding habits of my client's dogs, I have been able to observe and discover the fascinating relationship between diet, health and disease.

All those clients who have had sufficient faith in my ideas to try them with their own dogs. Their names would fill this book, so I shall be fair to all and single out none - with one exception. Thank you Clarissa Starrenburgh. Your early support and enthusiasm did much to keep me pushing forward and learning about nutrition, and better ways to feed dogs.

My clients in Lithgow for their ready acceptance of me and my ideas, and also for having cheerfully tolerated my many absences whilst this book was being completed.

Les Hart, without whom this book would not exist at all. It was Les who made it possible for me to stay at University and complete my veterinary training.

Kerrie Stanton who pushed me towards acupuncture, where I met Sharon Dart who introduced me to the idea of natural feeding of dogs. Thank you Sharon.

Paul Koller for numerous discussions, encouragement and for "focus".

Professor Robert W. Kirk, Professor of Medicine, Emeritus, New York State College of Veterinary Medicine, Cornell University, Ithaca New York, who was visiting Professor at Sydney University Veterinary School in 1974. One particular piece of advice he gave we aspiring veterinarians has had an enormous impact on the shape of my thinking, and subsequently, on this book. He advised us to ask the owners of healthy dogs, what those dogs were fed. This I have done, but I have extended that question to include the owners of unhealthy dogs as well. That suggestion, that question, and the subsequent answers are the foundations on which this book is built.

Dr. Dix Hawke for her early help, invaluable information, advice and encouragement.

Dr. Andrew Thompson for "vetting" and "doctoring" the section on Hydatidosis.

The many vets who have tried my ideas, found that they worked, and then pushed their own clients in that direction. In this respect, I particularly want to thank Drs. Vicki Higgins, Fiona Phillips, Bill Hood and Ross Perry.

The Post Graduate Committee in Veterinary Science at Sydney University for providing much of the solid scientific information re the major problems with commercial pet foods. Thank you Dr. Douglas Bryden for your support.

Dr. Tom Lonsdale for sharing your vision and having the courage to continue pushing for honesty, integrity and truth in our profession, in the face of strong opposition.

Elizabeth Shearman for her encouragement and editing skills.

ACKNOWLEDGEMENTS

Barry Willis for his invaluable input.

My family for their support and encouragement, in particular, to Dad for showing me integrity and persistence, to Mum, who instilled the concept of balance through variety, the place of imprecision and the importance of nutrition, to Elva Lennon, my "other mum" — for all sorts of reasons and for being there, to Roy and Margaret Castell, and their dogs Shambles, Guinevere, James and Penny, for their invaluable support, encouragement and assistance over the years, to Cathy for being herself, to Jackie a very special thanks for her cartoons which are scattered throughout the text and on the cover.

Finally to Elizabeth, for her criticism, support, photography, proof reading and her ownership of many problem animals.

How To Use this Book

My advice to you is - read it. The best way to read it is like a novel. From the beginning. Do that and you will most readily understand that raising healthy dogs is simple, cheap and uncomplicated.

However, if your dog is old - for example - you may wish to start with the last chapter. That is fine, but you will probably find it necessary to refer back to earlier chapters in order to have a full understanding of what I am saying. I often start at the end of books and work my way backwards. Have a look at the table of contents and decide what interests you.

After you have had a look at the contents page, glance through the chapters and note the headings on the pages. Those headings will give you a good idea of the topics covered in that chapter.

You will not find an index in this book. It is not a text book where you "look things up". For many people, the thoughts and the concepts I am conveying are new. They are a departure from stereotype veterinary thoughts. That is why I urge you to read the lot. Feel free to mark sections with a pen or a highlighter if you want to come back to them later - for whatever reason. Remember, books are to be used, not just left lying on a shelf.

Please enjoy,

Ian Billinghurst.

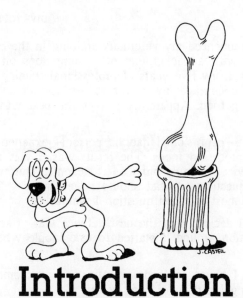

Introduction

This is a book about feeding dogs. It will show you in simple language ......

- How easy it is to feed dogs.
- How to feed your dog for maximum lifelong health.
- How to save money on dog food and help protect our environment.

You will learn how to use bones, food scraps and other food items, cheaply available from your local supermarket to produce a bright, active happy dog, with a minimum of health worries.

It also challenges a widespread belief that dogs should eat processed dog food. A belief that dog nutrition is a dead issue. That the dog food companies have made the need for a book such as this totally unnecessary.

Thirty years ago this book would not have been necessary. Thirty years ago, Australian dogs were fed on bones and leftovers. Everybody knew how to do it. It was common sense. As a consequence, most Australian dogs were very healthy.

That method of feeding dogs is now lost knowledge for many dog owners. It disappeared in the mid 60's when processed dog food became popular in Australia. In America that knowledge had largely disappeared by the mid-thirties.

When I commenced my veterinary training in the early seventies, I did so with a background of feeding dogs on bones and scraps. However, my five years of professional training taught me that I should encourage my clients to use scientifically balanced commercial dog food. Apparently it was the best way to feed a dog.

This lead to confusion. I had no personal experience of feeding dogs on processed foods. The result was, I was never quite sure what advice, I should hand out to clients. This was difficult because the question - "what should I feed my dog ?" - turned out to be the most common question I was asked.

However, I decided that the best defence was attack, and turned the question around. I started to ask people what they fed their dogs.

Meantime, I began to feed my own dogs on commercial dog food, something I had never done before.

Over a period of about two years, my formerly healthy dogs began to suffer numerous problems. Nothing major at first, but it was obvious that big trouble was looming. At first it was minor skin problems, runny eyes, scurfy coats, annoying itches, sore ears, anal sac problems, smelly coats, smelly faeces, smelly mouths, dental problems, the need for constant worming etc. However, with time it became reproductive problems and growth problems.

The embarrassing thing was that my own dogs for the first time ever, were suffering exactly the same sort of problems as my clients' dogs !

For me, this was a new experience. Before I became a vet I lived in the country where our dogs lived on a steady diet of rabbits, raw bones, and table scraps.

Back then, my dogs were neither wormed nor vaccinated. They became pregnant with no problems, and gave birth with ease to large litters. They were healthy dogs with a minimum of fuss.

However, all those health problems my dogs were developing, did tie in with the answers I was given when I questioned people concerning what they fed their dogs. I discovered that most people had exactly the same experience. Those who fed commercial dog food, had dogs with problems. Those who fed mostly bones and scraps had healthy dogs.

Over a period of eighteen years in small animal practice I have continued to ask that same question. I have asked the owners of both sick and healthy dogs what those dogs eat. The answers remain the same. Most of the sick dogs are fed either commercial dog food or badly designed home cooked food, while the really healthy dogs eat raw meaty bones, plus healthy food scraps.

Looking back on my experience with commercial dog food, I find it interesting that it took me as long as it did to realise what was happening. However, when I did, it did not take me long to make some changes.

In an attempt to do the very best by my dogs, and return them to a more common sense method of dog feeding, I began to read about so called "natural diets". It soon became obvious that the natural diets I was reading about were in essence, what I had always fed dogs. Bones, and healthy food scraps.

The bulk of their diet became raw meaty bones including lamb and raw chicken. The rest was mainly table scraps including left over vegetables, gravy, scraps of meat, fruit and small amounts of cereals such as rice, mashed potatoes and pasta. We added eggs, liver, kidneys, vegetable oils, honey, brewers yeast, kelp powder, cod liver oil and occasionally vitamin supplements.

I encouraged my clients to do the same.

This New Diet Saw Brilliant Health

An incredible change occured in all dogs fed the new diet.

No more skin problems, dental problems, eye problems, growth problems, reproductive problems etc etc. Less need for worming. Their faeces were less smelly and there was less of them. Their breath became, pleasant. Feeding them was cheaper, both in the cost of the food, and because they no longer needed expensive drugs or dentistry.

Over a period of two or three years I observed the results of many feeding trials carried out by myself and my clients. They all made the same basic statement.

Raw meaty bones promote health in dogs. Processed foods and cooked foods do not.

I began to realise that most of the disease problems we vets see are caused by only one thing - POOR NUTRITION.

The question I asked myself was .. "what is wrong with cooked and processed foods ? Why are bone eating dogs so healthy ?"

I have spent the last eight or nine years seeking answers to those questions.

This book is the culmination of a long process of seeking, learning, observing, reading, interrogating, researching and doing. There are numerous well researched reasons why commercial dog food fares so poorly in the dog health stakes, and why the raw meaty bones approach works so well. Explaining all of that is what much of this book is about.

More importantly, I have discovered that.....

Feeding Dogs is so Terribly Easy

Most modern dog owners are taught to believe that feeding dogs is such a difficult task, it is best left to the dog food companies. Nothing could be further from the truth. If you can get hold of a regular supply of raw meaty bones, you will have no problems whatsoever.

In fact feeding dogs can be explained in two or three lines. "Feed your dog a diet consisting of about sixty percent raw meaty bones. The rest of the diet should consist of a wide range of good quality human food scraps. Most of them should also be raw."

If you follow that advice, you cannot help but succeed. Your dog will be healthy, long-lived and happy. Not only that, you will save money with markedly reduced pet food costs, and a similar saving in veterinary bills.

What You Will Find in This Book

Chapters 1 - 4 deal with the nutritional dilemma facing modern dogs. You will learn why most modern dog foods produce ill health, poor performance, difficulty in reproducing and short lives.

Chapters 5 to 16 examine the commonly available food items which can be used to make and keep a dog healthy. The vital role of bones is explained, together with the use of vitamin supplements.

Chapters 17 - 22 talk about the practical feeding of normal healthy dogs.

The whole emphasis of the book is to show in a very practical way how easy it is to feed dogs for maximum health and longevity using low cost commonly available food items, many of which are currently used to either make poor quality dog food, or simply thrown away.

This approach to feeding your dog is healthier for your dog, your pocket and dare I say it - for our environment.

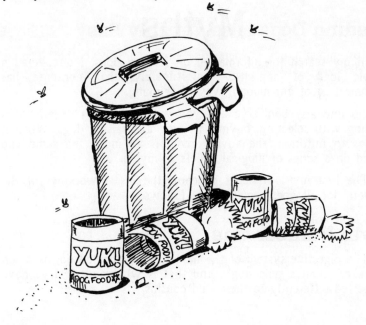

- 1 -

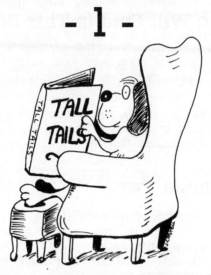

Modern Dog Feeding Myths

In my search for information on feeding dogs, I discovered a whole load of nonsense. Unfortunately, that nonsense has become part of our modern way of thinking.

Go into any bookstore and you will find half a dozen books dealing with selecting, buying, training and raising dogs. When it comes to nutrition, the advice given is all much the same and based on a series of illogical beliefs or myths.

The first myth or belief concerns the inside workings of the modern dog. It goes something as follows.....

Myth Number One

The digestive system of the modern domesticated dog is much "weaker" than a wild dog's, and that is why modern dogs have to be fed differently to their wild cousins.

That belief is based on nothing other than opinion. There have been no scientific studies to back it up.

On the contrary, the experiences of both scientists and numerous dog owners the world over confirm that the internal workings, including the entire digestive system, and the way food is utilised for growth, maintenance, repair and reproduction, is fundamentally the same in all dogs, both wild and domesticated.

Partly on the basis of that supposedly weaker metabolism in the modern dog, which in many people's minds includes their teeth, there have developed two further myths.....

Myth Number Two

Dogs should NOT eat bones, and.....

Myth Number Three

All dog food should be COOKED.

Unfortunately these ideas are self-perpetuating. Dogs fed cooked and processed food and no bones will always develop a weakened immune system and poor dental health.

The next myth, number four suggests that the intelligence of the modern dog owner has declined at about the same pace and degree as the modern dog's internal workings.

Myth Number Four

It is impossible without a university education in dog nutrition to be able to successfully feed a dog.

Because people have believed that modern dogs cannot be fed like wild dogs, they have attempted to feed dogs in all sorts of unnatural ways without bones. The results have often proved disasterous.

Those disasters have lead many people, including lots of vets to believe that feeding dogs is very difficult. This idea is reinforced by massive "education" campaigns launched by the major dog food companies.

Daily at meal times on television, weekly at dog shows, and monthly in various dog magazines, this message is reinforced in people's minds. "You cannot feed your dog properly.. but we can!" And so is born the next myth.....

Myth Number Five

The best way to feed a dog is with commercial dog food.

As if that were not bad enough, such a myth gives rise to myth number six.....

Myth Number Six

Each meal you feed to your dog should be complete and balanced.

On the face of it, that one sounds OK. However, it too, like the other five myths is a modern idea devised for no other reason than to enable the sale of pet foods. It has no scientific basis. On the contrary, it violates many natural feeding laws, and in the process lays the foundation for sick dogs.

Ask yourself the question... is that the way you design your own meals ? Each of them totally balanced with every conceivable nutrient present which you require ? Of course you don't. No creature since life began has eaten that way.

The attempt to put all the nutrients a dog requires in one product results in much ill-health. More of that shortly.

It is by reference to those six myths or beliefs that the majority of dog owners decide how their dog[s] should be fed. The result, as I have already mentioned, is a dog population which suffers numerous unnecessary and preventable health problems.

DEVELOPING A VALID APPROACH TO FEEDING DOGS

I would like to develop with you, a new set of beliefs on which to base scientific and healthy methods of feeding dogs.

To do that, I will re-state the first myth, the one that claims the internal workings of dogs have declined dramatically since they were domesticated.

It now becomes .....

Fact Number One

Although the mind and the outward appearance of our modern dog has changed dramatically, the internal workings, including the entire digestive system, and the way food is utilised for growth, maintenance, repair and reproduction, is fundamentally the same as it's wild ancestors.

- If that is so, a study of the foods eaten by wild dogs, should provide us with a sound basis for feeding modern dogs.

ASKING THE DOG ABOUT FEEDING DOGS

There are six words which may be used to describe the eating habits of a wolf and other wild dogs. Those words are carnivore, hunter, scavenger, opportunist, vegetarian and omnivore.

Each of those words has great significance when it comes to deciding what our modern domestic dog can and ought to eat. Let's start off with the word carnivore.

Your Dog is a Carnivore

Dogs, like wolves love to eat other animals. They will eat their internal organs, their meat, their bones, everything. I am talking about all dogs. It does not matter whether you own a chihuahua, a maltese, a great dane, a poodle or a bull terrier-cross-rottweiler. They all love to eat this way.

The fact that a dog is able and loves to eat meat, bones, and internal organs etc. makes your dog a carnivore.

That means all of those different parts of an animal's carcase can and should, form part of your dog's balanced diet.

Your Dog is a Vegetarian

The wolf and other wild dogs are also vegetarians. One of the first things eaten by a wild dog when it kills, are the stomach and intestinal contents. These contain fermenting grass and similar plant materials.

Wild dogs and modern dogs love to eat over-ripe fruit of all different kinds. They scavenge round the bottom of fruit trees. They dine regularly at the compost heap.

WARNING: Do not put corn cobs or cooked bones into compost heaps to which dogs have access - both can cause obstructions.

Many modern dog owners tell me how their dogs actually fight over fruit.

During the second world war in Europe, many dogs survived and reproduced successfully on the stomach contents of sheep and cattle. Their health was reported as outstanding.

What this means is that both fruit and vegetables should be part of a balanced diet for modern dogs. The fruit is usually best if it is over-ripe, and the vegetables should be pulverised until they resemble the gut contents of an animal such as a sheep or a rabbit or a deer etc. More of that in chapter ten.

Your Dog is a Scavenger

Your dog is a scavenger. You only have to leave your dog alone with an open garbage can to find that out.

Dogs will eat and derive food value from practically anything. To a wild dog, soil eating is an important source of minerals. Bark from trees is an important source of fibre.

As scavengers or cleaner-uppers, wild dogs eat the left-overs from every animal that is killed or dies. This means wild dogs eat lots of bones which means your dog is adapted to eat, and actually requires to eat, if it is to remain in good health, lots of bones.

Dogs receive valuable nutrients from material that we humans find totally repugnant. Things like vomit, faeces and decaying flesh.

I constantly see farm dogs fight over the stinking rotten infected remains of a cow's afterbirth.

A colleague of mine who regularly autopsies pigs told me that his dogs live almost entirely on raw pig bits, including the internal organs etc. His dogs are brilliantly healthy. He did assure me that they were wormed regularly.

Dogs also eat faeces. This habit is called "Coprophagy". It may seem a revolting habit, but for dogs, it is perfectly normal.

They obviously like it, but what benefit do dogs derive from eating faeces ? Faeces are a highly valuable food, consisting of the dead and living bodies of millions upon millions of bacteria.

This makes faeces an excellent source of very high quality protein, of essential fatty acids, fat soluble vitamins, particularly vitamin K, the whole range of B vitamins, many different minerals because of the soil in it, and a host of other nutritional factors including anti-oxidants and enzymes and also valuable fibre.

Many dogs that eat commercial dog food, particularly the dry dog food, have to eat faeces to stay healthy. Usually their own. Cat's droppings are also very popular. The faeces they eat is of far greater benefit to them than the product produced by the dog food companies.

Your dog needs to be fed faeces and similar revolting material or their equivalent if it is to remain healthy.

If you do not want your dog to eat faeces, and people who kiss their dogs usually don't, then you must provide in the diet all those nutrients which are currently missing from your dog's diet, and which faeces supplies.

To replace faeces requires a team of ingredients like yoghurt, brewers yeast, eggs, polyunsaturated oils, an enzyme supplement and crushed raw vegetables as a source of fibre.

Your Dog is a Hunter

This means your dog also enjoys fresh food of animal origin. Dogs will eat anything that moves. This starts at a very young age with insects, beetles, ants, lizards, whatever walks or crawls or slithers into it's path.

As time passes, birds and small mammals are tackled. Later on, with the help of other dogs, larger prey such as deer, sheep, goats, cattle etc. are eaten.

Your Dog is an Opportunist

This means that a hungry dog will take the opportunity to eat whatever food is available.

That is why dogs will survive and do well on an all fruit and vegetable diet, the ruminal contents of cows, sheep etc., on a carnivorous diet of whole animals, or whatever.

Many dogs survive happily on the contents of garbage cans. This has prompted many a client to ask me ... "Why is it that my dog with the best of modern food and modern medical attention gets sick while those dogs which roam the streets never seem to get a thing wrong with them ?"

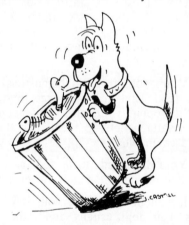

The answer is simple. A dog roaming the streets, seeking out it's own food, is living closer to nature and the lifestyle designed for it by evolution, than the majority of pampered pooches. It may not have the same foods it's ancestors had to choose from, but at the same time it is not limited by what some human or dog food company chooses for it. It has a much wider choice. Much of the food is raw, including vegetable peelings, rotten fruit and some bones. It gets plenty of the right sort of exercise. Purposeful exercise in the pursuit of food or whatever it chooses to do.

Your Dog is an Omnivore

The fact that your dog is a carnivore, a vegetarian, a scavenger, a hunter and an opportunist means that your dog is an omnivore.

This means a dog can eat practically anything in the way of food. In fact so far as eating goes, your dog is one of the most versatile creatures on earth.

Keep this word in mind when you are trying to decide whether or not you should feed a particular food to a dog. Many people say to me ... "I did not think you were... supposed .... able... to feed such and such to a dog." The truth is, whatever you can feed other animals can usually be fed to dogs. Whatever you can safely feed to humans may be fed to dogs.

Man and dog are both omnivores, but with totally opposite backgrounds. The dog is an omnivore with a carnivorous background, while human beings are omnivores with a vegetarian/ fruitarian background.

That is why a dog has the teeth and body of a carnivore, while humans have the teeth and body of a vegetable and fruit eater, but we both have the internal workings of an omnivore.

This ability to eat similar foods is why the dog has remained a companion of man for so long. The dog will survive on just about anything we care to throw at it, even commercial dog food !

WHAT HAVE WE LEARNT FROM THOSE WILD DOGS ?

The first and most obvious fact is that.....

The Dog is a Bone Eater

We must conclude that not only do dogs eat bones, but that because raw meaty bones form the basis of the diet of wild dogs, they should also form the basis of the diet of modern domestic dogs.

Dogs Eat Offal

Liver, kidneys, heart, lungs, brains etc are all part of the diet of a wild dog. If they are available, they too should form part of the diet devised for modern dogs.

Dogs Eat Vegetable Material

Sometimes in vast quantities, as when they eat the guts of a cow. They also eat fruit. Usually over ripe fruit. All the vegetables they eat are crushed, finely divided and raw. What they have never eaten in vast quantities, is something we modern humans pour down their throats by the truckload, cooked grain.

Dogs Eat all Sorts of Rotten and Revolting Food

This includes such things as faeces, vomit, after-birth, rotten meat etc.. This material is often full of micro-organisms, commonly known as "germs". This means that what we feed the modern dog should contain the nutrients present in those rotten "germy" foods. Brewers yeast and yoghurt help.

Dogs Eat Fresh Raw Food

Everybody knows that dogs eat fresh foods as well as rotten foods. However, there is a big question about raw food. The fact that dogs can and will eat raw food is so self evident it hardly needs stating, and yet, it is such a controversial issue, I discuss it at some length in the next chapter.

Dogs Achieve a Balanced Diet Over a Period of Time

Wild dogs eat what they can when they can. Because of this variety, over a period of time they achieve balance and completeness. Is that the way we should feed modern dogs ?

Is it better to achieve balance at every meal, or is it better to do as nature does, achieve balance through a series of meals ?

Common sense and experience tells me that nature may well be correct. In our dog feeding programme using bones and other natural products, we have never attempted to achieve balance at every meal. I am pleased to report brilliant health in our dogs.

On the other hand, I have uncovered a lot of evidence to

suggest that by lumping all the components of a balanced diet together as do the dog food companies, and the people who prepare "stews" for their dogs, we cause a wide range of health problems. [See chapter 6]

That Leaves us with Four Questions Still to Answer:

- Firstly, can a modern person feed a dog without a higher degree in dog nutrition ?

You will soon realise how easy it is to feed dogs, so forget about that concern.

- Secondly, what about commercial dog food ? Is it better than a dog's natural diet ?

I suspect you know the answer to that one. However, if you are still not convinced, I am confident you will be after reading chapter three where I discuss in detail the pros and cons of commercial dog food.

- Thirdly, food cooked or raw .. which is best ?

The answer is raw, but do read Chapter 2 for more details.

- Fourthly, how can we know our dog's diet is balanced ?

That too will become clear as you read on.

By a careful consideration of the above you should be able to discover some guiding principles to use in feeding dogs. I have pulled out four of them. You can use those principles to make the feeding of dogs very simple, cheap and health promoting.

Principle Number One

- A dog's diet should be based on raw meaty bones.

Principle Number Two

- Most of a dog's diet should be raw.

Principle Number Three

● Apart from raw meaty bones, a dog should be fed on as wide a variety of foods as possible, and those foods should reflect the types and quantities of foods wild dogs eat.

Principle Number Four

● Instead of attempting to feed a dog all the nutrients it needs at each and every meal, the diet should be balanced over many different meals. The reasons for this will become clear as you read on.

These are the principles I shall use to develop healthy dietary programmes for dogs. However, before doing that, I need to talk about the various food items commonly available, that may be used to feed dogs.

In the next two chapters I discuss two questions raised in this chapter, the question of cooked vs raw food, and the question of the problems associated with processed foods.

- 2 -

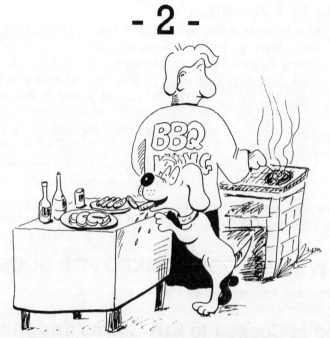

The Question of Cooked or Raw Foods ?

- Most people are very confused about this. They hear conflicting advice from many quarters. Most commonly they are advised to cook their dog's food. Rarely are they told why.

People Cook Their Dog's Food for all Sorts of Reasons.

- One is so their dog will not take baits. Unfortunately many baits are given with cooked food.
- Others believe that dogs are "supposed" to eat cooked food. Somebody told them, or they "heard" it somewhere.
- Often the food is cooked "to prevent worms or distemper or... something ..... ?"
- Some people cannot cope with their dog eating raw meat and offal.
- Many cook their dog's food because they believe it will become more nutritious and more easily digested.

Most people admit they have no idea at all what they should do. Sometimes they feed it raw and sometimes they feed it cooked.

SO WHY IS FOOD COOKED FOR DOGS ?

There are some very good reasons why food is cooked.

Food is Cooked to Kill Germs and the Toxins They Produce

If there are any dangerous germs in your dog's food, proper cooking will destroy them.

Cooking Your Dog's Food Kills any Parasites

Cooking prevents the transfer of parasites from the dog's food to humans. Particularly the hydatid tapeworm. Hydatidosis is a potentially fatal disease which can be transmitted to man from various animals including sheep, pigs, kangaroos, wallabys, cattle etc..

For more information on this problem please read Chapter 9, where raw foods and the hydatid problem are discussed.

Food is Cooked so it can be Stored and Transported

Raw food "goes off" or self-destructs due to the activity of it's own enzymes.

Cooking stops this process by destroying the enzymes. This allows food to be transported and stored.

Food is Cooked to Make it More Nutritious and More Digestible

Is that a valid reason ? In general .. no. There are exceptions to this. Grains and certain vegetables require to be cooked for various reasons, but in most cases cooking food does not make it any more digestible or nutritious.

Cooking physically breaks food down, making it more easily "got at" by your dog's digestive enzymes. This includes meat and vegetables.

Apart from that digestive aid, cooking does nothing to make food more nutritious. In fact cooked food for a variety of reasons loses much of it's nutritive value.

It is popularly supposed that dogs cannot digest raw vegetables. However, if raw vegetables are physically broken down such as with a food processor or a juicer, your dog can easily digest them.

DESTRUCTIVE EFFECTS OF COOKING

Cooking Destroys Vitamins

Heat destroys many vitamins. Particularly a number of the B vitamins and vitamin C. Many are lost with the cooking water.

Cooking Destroys Enzymes

All living tissue contains enzymes in abundance. Enzymes are proteins which control the chemical reactions which in their totality, constitute the life of an animal. Those enzymes are destroyed by heat.

The enzymes in raw food are now recognised as important nutrients. As nutrients they have two basic functions:

Firstly, they aid the digestion of the food they are found in, and secondly they help slow the ageing process.

The destruction of enzymes in food forces the pancreas to work harder. It has to produce more digestive enzymes. The result is several diseases in dogs, including Pancreatitis, Pancreatic Insufficiency and sugar Diabetes. Closely linked with this problem is the poor availability of zinc in modern processed foods, particularly the dried dog foods.

Enzymes in food are absorbed whole into the bloodstream. Once in the body, they help slow and even reverse the damaging effects of a process in the body called "cross-linking". Cross-linking is one of the most damaging of the ageing effects. It causes skin to become wrinkled and inelastic, arteries to become hard and brittle, and is one of the mechanisms by which the molecules found in genes become damaged, resulting in cancer and birth deformities.

In other words, by cooking your dog's food, you are contributing in no small way to your dog's ageing processes and in the case of stud dogs and bitches, you are contributing to reproductive problems.

Cooking Destroys Other Naturally Occuring Anti-Ageing Factors

Anti-ageing factors called anti-oxidants which are present in raw foods, are destroyed by cooking. That is why cooked food is less able to slow the ageing process, and is involved in all of the degenerative diseases of old age, including cancer, kidney disease, heart disease, arthritis etc., etc..

Cooking Can Reduce Protein Value and Availability

Excessive cooking results in proteins becoming indigestible. It also causes the loss of two essential amino acids. Lysine and methionine. That loss results in growth problems, bone problems, skin problems problems in pregnancy, milk production, and general poor health and reduced resistance to disease.

Cooking Produces "Foreign" Foods

When food is cooked, the fats, the proteins, the carbohydrates, that is, all the major nutrients are changed. The greater the degree of cooking, the greater the changes. The greater the changes, the more indigestible that food becomes. Also, the more the body regards such molecules as foreign.

These foreign chemicals can result in allergic reactions, including auto-immune diseases like arthritis. Many of these "new chemicals" are carcinogenic or cancer forming.

In other words, modern cooked foods, such as commercial dog foods, not only lack many protective nutrients [vitamins, enzymes, anti-oxidants and other anti-ageing factors], but also are full of dangerous chemicals which actively promote cancer and other degenerative diseases.

No Teeth Cleaning and No Exercise Required to Eat it.

A dog subjected to a lifetime of cooked food is deprived of chewing, ripping and tearing at food. This means that an important aspect of the food as creating exercise for a dog is lost. It also means that a dog's teeth are not cleaned. That in itself creates major health problems for the dog as infected and decaying teeth send toxins and bacteria throughout it's body.

Cooking Food Makes it More Tasty ... Sounds Great ?

Cooked food tastes and smells a whole lot better than raw food. This is true for most people and most dogs.

The question is, have we gained anything for our dogs by making their food more palatable ?

The only time palatability is useful, is when you are trying to coax a sick dog to commence eating. Apart from that one advantage, not much has been gained. The major problem is that cooked food is addictive. This leads to a number of problems.

- ● LOSS OF INSTINCT TO CHOOSE

Dogs eating a raw, whole food diet, are usually able to use instinct to make suitable choices if presented with a sufficiently wide variety of foods. Modern cooked food abolishes this natural instinct because of it's addictive effects.

- ● THE CREATION OF AN UNBALANCED DIET

Dogs fed cooked food often train their owner to feed them a narrow range of favourites. This always leads to an unbalanced diet with health problems being the inevitable consequence.

- ● DIFFICULTY IN CHANGING DIETS

It can be difficult but not impossible to change the eating habits of older animals raised on cooked food.

- ● OBESITY

Because cooked food tastes so good, over-eating and hence obesity is common.

- ● IT HELPS SELL THOSE AWFUL PET FOODS

Pet food companies, use the addictive qualities of cooked food to help sell their product. People buy food which their dog likes.

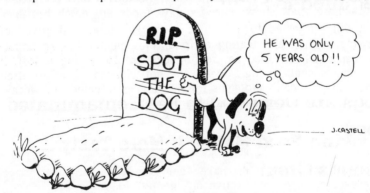

SPOT THE DOG WHO ATE COOKED
FOOD ALL HIS LIFE.

The Bottom Line on Cooked Food

When food is cooked, it retains sufficient nutrients to keep your dog alive with no obvious immediate problems. It does not however allow your dog to have a long, healthy, trouble-free life. It is responsible for much ill health including cancer, kidney disease, heart disease, arthritis, pancreatic disease etc. In short, dogs fed on cooked foods live shorter, less healthy, more miserable lives.

DOES THAT MEAN OUR DOGS SHOULD EAT RAW FOODS ?

Wild dogs live exclusively on raw foods. Their whole metabolism is geared to the consumption of raw foods. Modern dogs are no different which is sufficient justification for feeding them in exactly the same way.

However, many folk require a lot more evidence before they will feed their dogs raw food. Let's examine that evidence.

The Results of Feeding Trials

The most tangible evidence is the numerous results of feeding trials. Those trials show dogs fed raw foods are much healthier than dogs fed cooked foods.

Modern dogs fed on processed food and home cooked foods have weaker immune systems, and they age more quickly.

Dogs are Designed to Eat Contaminated Food

Many people are worried by the "germs" in raw food. They believe those germs will make their dog sick. However, dogs have evolved to eat and thrive on "germy" food.

Your dog being a scavenger, thrives on the presence of microbes in his or her food. Wild dogs eat the gut contents of their prey, and the faeces of many different animals. They also eat soil, contaminated meat, buried bones, infected meat and so on. These are all a source of microbes and any toxins they might produce.

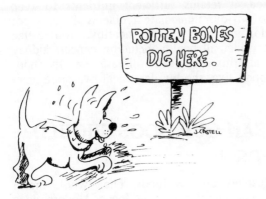

These microbe contaminated foods are a rich source of a wide range of healthy nutrients for a dog including proteins, fatty acids, enzymes, anti-oxidants and vitamins etc.. Dogs are designed to eat this type of food !

Raw Offal can be Safely Eaten

Raw offal is part of a dog's natural diet, and is full of valuable nutrients. The bottom line here is that lamb and lamb offal from your butcher is quite safe. If in doubt consider the use of raw chicken offal in your healthy dog feeding programme. See Chapter 9 for details on offal.

Dogs Depend upon Enzymes in Raw Foods

For millions of years, dogs have relied on the enzymes present in their food to help with the digestive process.

Cooked food does not have those enzymes. On the other hand, food which is mechanically broken down without heating retains all it's enzymes and is actually more easily digested than cooked food.

That is why your dog can actually digest raw vegetables better than cooked vegetables. All you have to do is physically break up those vegetables before feeding them to your dog.

For more information on feeding raw vegetables to your dog, see Chapter 10.

CONCLUSION

In other words, it is important to feed your dog on fresh RAW wholesome food. This principle is the reason I cannot recommend some of the supposedly better dog foods currently available. The ones marketed by newcomers to the pet food industry, who claim to use top quality ingredients. These foods which I cannot name for obvious reasons, being a cooked product, have all the drawbacks of cooked foods.

HANDLING RAW FOODS

Naturally, for the sake of our own health we always make sure that the raw food we feed to our dogs in no way contaminates our own food.

If using kitchen utensils to prepare dog food, take all the same precautions you would normally take when handling raw foods for your own consumption. That includes near-boiling water for cleaning, proper washing and drying etc.

STORING RAW FOODS

Store them in exactly the same way you would store food for yourself in order to preserve maximum nutrition. That is, refrigerate meat and bones, or freeze them if buying in bulk and storing for longer periods; refrigerate vegetables and so on.

Frozen food has in general less nutritional value than fresh food, but in our experience is far more health promoting than food preserved by cooking.

Also note that the wolf, your dog's ancestor has a long history of eating frozen meat and bones. This is the way many wolves survive their winter. In other words, the wolf, and therefore your dog, is actually adapted by long evolution to use frozen food as a normal part of it's diet.

- It is strongly advised that from the point of view of human health, you store your refrigerated and frozen raw dog foods separately from the family's foods.

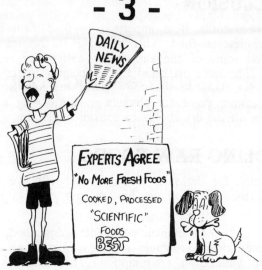

Knowing Your Enemy is Half the Battle - Commercial Dog Food

If you know all about the food value of commercial dog foods, please move on to the next chapter. If you think processed foods are the best way to feed dogs, it would be worthwhile to keep reading.

What follows is not an exhaustive treatment of the subject of commercial dog food. That in itself would take many books. It is a summary of some of the relevant facts I have learned about these products. I have no doubt, that with the passage of time, many problems, other than the ones I mention in connection with them will be discovered.

A SHORT HISTORY OF DOG FOOD

Commercial dog food was first manufactured in the 1850's in England. It was a biscuit type product, based on cereals and meat meal.

In 1885 the idea caught on in the States. Astute mill owners realised the huge profit potential in feeding the nation's dogs on the scraps of their industry. Their dog food was composed of milling by-products, the floor-sweepings, plus meat-meal. The modern product has not changed substantially.

In 1922, Ken-L-Ration, which was canned horse meat, hit the market in the States. This has since been followed by many other types of canned dog food.

Commercial dog food is now the most popular method of feeding dogs in Australia, America and Great Britain. That is why vets are commonly asked "...which dog food is the best ? Which one should I feed my dog ?" This chapter is here to help answer that question. I hope it helps you decide not to feed any of them.

Dogs have lived, reproduced and been extremely healthy without commercial dog food for millions of years. It is only in the last thirty years that Australian dogs have eaten these products in large volumes. In that period their general health has declined dramatically.

AUSTRALIAN DOGS USED TO BE PRETTY HEALTHY

As a veterinary student in the early seventies, I found it hard to understand why Aussie vets had fewer and simpler dog and cat diseases to deal with than the Americans. It seemed to make the Aussie vet somehow inferior. We did not need to be trained to the same high degree of complexity and sophistication.

There was a simple explanation. At that time, more than

seventy percent of Aussie dogs were still fed bones and scraps. They were still pretty healthy.

American dogs had been eating processed food and no bones for decades. They had developed a wide range of problems. Their vets had had to develop a complex set of diagnostic and thera-peutic tools to deal with them.

I need not have worried. Our dogs' disease problems are in-creasing on a par with their increasing consumption of processed and cooked foods. We Aussie vets now have to be as good as our American counterparts to deal with them.

The question in many people's minds, the question I have been seeking answers to for some years is why ?

WHY DO PROCESSED FOODS CAUSE PROBLEMS ?

There are a multitude of reasons. It all begins with the reason that dog food exists.

Dog Food Does Not Exist to Make Dogs Healthy

Dog food manufacturers take useless wastes from the human food industry and sell it as dog food. Why do they bother ? Advertising implies they are there to promote the health of dogs. Their primary concern is in fact profit.

The laws which govern dog food production do not require it to promote health, reproduction, growth, or longevity. The law requires that it contains specified minimal amounts of certain nutrients. So long as the product meets those requirements the law is satisfied.

A careful examination of dog food advertising shows that most manufacturers make no claim that their product promotes best health, best growth, best working capacity, best reproductive ability, or longevity and freedom from disease.

What they will claim is that the product contains certain nutrients which meet it's legal obligations. In their advertise-ments, they allow dog owners to make claims about the product for them, or they refer to some aspect of the product which people assume is associated with good nutrition and good health. All this is done in such a way that people make favourable assumptions about the product which are not necessarily true.

Unfortunately, they have even conned people who claim to be vets into endorsing these products.

Processed Food Loses Nutritional Value

All processed foods lose much of their nutritional value by the various processing methods involved. This may prompt you to ask...

"So why is it done ? Why is food processed if it becomes less valuable nutritionally as a result ? "

If food is not processed, it will not keep. It will go off. In other words, the main reason food is processed, is to enable it to be stored and transported without deteriorating.

FRESH FOOD SPOILS BECAUSE -
- It's own enzymes break it down.
- It combines with oxygen.
- It is attacked by micro-organisms.

To prevent this happening, the makers of commercial food products have to REMOVE the enzyme rich parts of some foods. Most foods have to be COOKED in order to destroy any

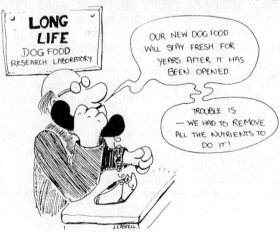

enzymes, together with parasites and micro-organisms. Sometimes the food is preserved with ADDED CHEMICALS including salt, sugar, and many others, and then packaged to exclude oxygen and "germs".

Unfortunately, all this processing removes or destroys the nutrients that promote health and prevent disease. This includes enzymes, vitamins, and natural anti-oxidants. Added chemicals such as salt and sugar actively promote poor health.

EACH FORM OF DOG FOOD HAS IT'S PROBLEMS

Dry Dog Foods

Dry dog food is the cheapest commercially produced dog food available. The cost is about one half to one third the cost of feeding canned dog food. It is the most popular form of dog food in the United States. In Australia, the most popular way to feed a dog is on a mixture of canned and dry dog food.

Dry dog foods are made from cereals and cereal by-products plus meat by-products composed of ground up cooked bone and offal. To this is added fat, vitamins and minerals. They contain about 10 % water.

Dry dog foods are low in digestibility and nutritional value. They are made from low quality ingredients which have undergone an extremely harsh form of cooking. They are low in energy, fats, good quality protein, most vitamins and many minerals. They contain lots of starch and calcium.

Dry dog food is supposed to prevent tartar build up on the teeth because of it's abrasive effect. Numerous controlled studies demonstrate that this is not true. Most promote almost as much tartar build up as canned food.

Because dry dog foods are low in energy, poorly digested and high in insoluble fibre, they result in very moist, offensive and voluminous stools. Those wet offensive stools result in a concentrated urine which burns the lawn. In addition the high levels of cereal products cause an alkaline urine, high in certain minerals.

This combination helps produce both bladder stones and bladder infections.

The stones can make it difficult for your dog to urinate, or they reach enormous sizes in the bladder, causing discomfort, and the need for surgery or expensive diets to get rid of them.

Because of their low nutritional value, dry dog foods are unsuitable for growing, pregnant, lactating, working or thin dogs that need to gain weight.

If you wish to use a dry dog food for such purposes, find one formulated with extra nutrients. Only use it if controlled trials have demonstrated it's suitability for your purpose. Do not simply believe the advertised claims..... Good luck in your search.

The major consistent disadvantage of dry dog foods is that most of them are deficient in ESSENTIAL FATTY ACIDS. Essential fatty acids are an essential nutrient commonly found in plant oils and chicken or pork fat. Like vitamins they are essential for the proper functioning of your dog's body. Without sufficient of them in it's diet, your dog will develop a range of diseases,including problems with growth, reproduction and the most awful skin diseases.

This is a MAJOR FAULT with dry dog foods. It is why there are so many health problems, particularly skin problems and reproductive problems, in the canine world today.

The reproductive and skin problems caused by dry dog foods are also due to a lack of zinc. This is caused by the excessive calcium in most dry dog foods. The calcium combines with the zinc producing a compound which cannot be absorbed, resultng in a zinc deficiency.

This lack of zinc results in health problems at all stages of a dog's life. It is involved in skeletal and growth problems, skin problems, infertility of both sexes, sugar Diabetes, Pancreatitis, Pancreatic Insufficiency..... the list goes on and on.

The excessive calcium in dry dog foods is heavily implicated as a cause of bloat in the adult dog and of skeletal problems in growing dogs.

Dry dog foods have a short shelf life. The fats in them rapidly become rancid and they quickly lose vitamins. They must be stored under cool dry conditions. High temperature and high humidity hasten their deterioration.

If you must use dried dog foods, buy no more than a months supply, always purchase it from a place with a quick turnover and always check the "use by" date.

- Some people find their dogs will not eat it.
- My response is .... great.. sensible dog.

In summary, dry dog foods in Australia are cheap, moderately unpalatable dog foods that are low in nutritional value and cause numerous health problems in many dogs. Although very popular because of their cheapness and convenience, they are in general the very worst form of processed food.

Soft Moist Foods

These are intermediate in water content between canned food and dry food, containing about 30 % water. They are probably the least popular of all the commercial dog foods.

They look a bit like fresh meat patties or mincemeat or rissoles, depending on how they are presented and packaged . They do not require refrigeration, which certainly makes them convenient. They cost about the same as canned foods.

They are usually very palatable and high in energy. If fed free choice they will result in obesity. Their high energy content and supposed greater palatability implies that they may be useful in feeding a thin reluctant-to-eat animal, or an animal that requires extra energy, such as a pregnant animal, a lactating animal, or one exposed to the cold or doing lots of hard work etc..

However, I would not recommend them. They are high in energy because they contain large amounts of soluble carbohydrates including such things as corn syrup and a carbohydrate called propylene glycol. None of these "foods" have been part of a dog's evolutionary history.

Apart from supplying energy and making the food more palatable, these soluble carbohydrates act as preservatives. That is, because of their water retaining nature they prevent spoilage by bacteria and fungi.

The soft moist foods often contain acids such as hydrochloric, phosphoric or malic. These acids keep the pH low, which also helps to reduce spoilage.

Sometimes better quality ingredients, such as fresh animal tissues are used in their production. However, because of costs this is not usual. They are mostly made from much the same ingredients as dry dog foods which means they are able to produce similar problems, together with the added problems that a diet high in soluble carbohydrates brings. This includes such problems as obesity, sugar Diabetes and dental problems.

These products can hardly be recommended !

Canned Dog Foods

Canned dog foods in Australia contain about 80 % water. This is an expensive way to buy water. Due to clever marketing,

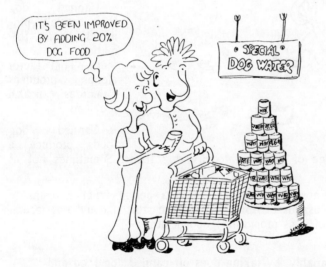

they are the most popular form of commercial dog food. This contrasts with America, where dry foods are the most popular.

It costs two to three times as much to feed canned food compared to dry dog food.

They are made from similar ingredients to dry dog foods, but usually contain less cereal and more animal tissue.

Dogs usually find them more palatable than dry dog foods. This is because of their higher fat, protein and water content.

They are higher in energy content and are usually more digestible than dry dog food. They have the longest shelf life of all the commercial dog foods.

In common with all commercial dog foods, a major factor involved in their purchase is that they are CONVENIENT.

The majority of people find that canned dog food is pretty revolting when opened. The "freshly" opened can smells very similar to the residue which leaves the dog at the other end.

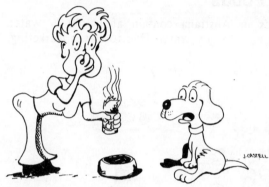

Canned dog food actively promotes tartar formation on the teeth. That factor alone produces numerous health problems.

Canned dog foods produce a similar range of problems to dry dog foods. Sometimes not as quickly.

Having observed over an 18 year period what happens to literally thousands of dogs that eat the stuff, I could not recommend any of it as promoting good health.

- Invariably, by taking dogs off canned dog food and switching them to a properly formulated diet based on raw meaty bones, their health improves immensely.

Additives in Dog Foods

It is widely believed that it is the additives in commercial dog foods, the colourings, the flavourings and the preservatives which are responsible for most of the ill health these products produce.

If only it were that simple. In some dogs, chemical additives do cause hypersensitivity reactions, allergies, skin problems, over activity etc. In fact most dogs eating the commercial products appear to "be overactive" to some degree.

- However, the vast majority of problems, which result from feeding commercially produced foods are caused by other faults.

Modern Dog Foods Cause Dental Problems

Bone eating Aussie dogs of the mid 1970's had very few dental problems. When dogs eat bones, when they rip and tear and crunch bones, their teeth and gums are exercised, cleaned and massaged. In addition, the stronger immune system of bone eating dogs adds to the health of the mouth.

Contrast that with today's non-bone-eating dog in which dental disease is reaching epidemic proportions. The foods eaten by dogs today, cooked and processed foods, are high in two substances; soluble carbohydrates and soluble calcium. Those two unusual [for a dog] nutrients, attack a dog's mouth at every meal. In addition, processed foods have no chance of cleaning teeth the way raw meaty bones do.

Look in your dog's mouth. Smell it ! What you see and what you smell depend on your dog's eating habits. Dogs that regularly eat bones have healthy mouths. The mouths of dogs that eat processed and cooked foods are definite "no-go" zones.

Veterinary dentistry is an increasing source of income for Australian vets as more dogs spend their lives eating processed foods and no bones. We even have a Veterinary Dentistry Association !

In the United States, where 90 % of dogs eat processed foods, more than a third of the income of the veterinary profession is derived from dentistry in pet animals.

By the time many modern dogs are 5 years old, their teeth

are covered with a thick crust of tartar. The gums are bleeding, infected and painful. Tartar is the mouth's attempt to repair tooth enamel. It is composed of calcium salts. High concentrations of calcium in modern dog foods contribute to excessive tartar formation.

Tartar formation begins within twenty minutes of eating. The tartar is home to millions of bacteria.

The bacteria in the tartar thrive on the soluble carbohydrates found in commercial dog food. They invade the gums, the tooth roots and the tooth enamel causing severe gum infection [gingivitis] and generalised mouth infections accompanied by tooth root decay, pain, difficulty in eating, rotten breath and eventually loss of teeth.

Most people are aware that canned dog food actively promotes tartar formation without removing it, but many think dry dog foods prevent tartar formation. They do not. The product is either gulped straight down, or it crumbles rapidly, or it quickly becomes wet. In any event, the supposed abrasive effect of this food is quickly lost. They also, like canned foods are high in both soluble carbohydrates and calcium.... a perfect recipe for tartar formation.

Small breeds are more commonly affected. Some people think maltese terriers have a genetic predisposition to bad teeth. They don't. It is just that the smaller breeds are more likely to be deprived of bones, particularly if they have long hair. These dogs often share their smelly mouth infections with their owners. This problem is easy to deal with in the dog, but I have never been game to tackle an owner about his or her problem!

Accompanying all of these dental problems in dogs is very poor health. This is because the bacteria responsible for the mouth infection, spread themselves and the toxins they produce throughout the body. These bacteria invade many organs and tissues, targeting most particularly the kidneys and the heart which can both become infected. This eventually contributes to both kidney and heart disease. However, any other organ can become infected by these blood borne bacteria, for example the lungs or the prostate in a male, or the lining of the womb in a female.

The bottom line is, the combination of no bones and commercial dog foods is devastating to the health of all pet dogs because of it's effect on dental health.

Unfortunately, that is not the end of the story.

The All Purpose Dog Food is a Poor Product

Australian dog foods are mostly "all-purpose products". That is, they are supposed to be able to be fed to a dog at any stage of it's life. This contrasts with the situation in America, where there are three different types of dog food.

- The first type is a MAINTENANCE food.

It is fed to sedentary non-growing and non-reproducing dogs. That is, household pets. Maintenance foods are designed to contain minimum amounts of all the essential nutrients. They are not supposed to have sufficient nutrients to support growth, reproduction or activity.

- The second type is a GROWTH food.

These foods are used to feed puppies and pregnant or nursing females. They are supposed to contain extra calories, protein, vitamins and minerals in sufficient quantities to support growth.

- The third type is a food designed for PERFORMANCE.

These are sold as food for dogs doing lots of hard work such as sled dogs, racing greyhounds, cattle dogs etc. Performance foods should contain extra energy to support the activities of these dogs.

- In Australia there are very few specific-purpose dog foods.

Most are said to be all-purpose products which supposedly can be used in any situation from puppies to adults, including pregnant dogs and old-age pensioner dogs.

This is not possible given the nature of commercial dog food which is forced to contain "a complete and balanced diet" in every can or bag. It is not possible because each stage of life has different nutrient requirements, and while it is possible to vary the proportions of fresh whole foods to suit those varying needs, this is not possible with a supposedly "scientifically balanced" food.

This is a major reason that they perform poorly in every one of those situations. The most obvious problem with this approach is the excessive levels of many nutrients. High levels of protein, minerals, and energy [calories] may be suitable for a young, growing and active dog, but hardly suitable for a sedentary, layabout house pet.

The net result is that many older pets suffer obesity, skin diseases and degenerative diseases associated with continual excesses of calories, salt, protein, phosphorus, and calcium.

Most Dog Foods Contain High Cereal Levels

Large amounts of cereals are completely unsuitable for dogs when fed as the bulk of their diet. Cooked cereals have not figured in a dog's evolutionary history. The result is that dogs raised on predominantly cereal diets, and this includes most dog foods, develop numerous health problems including such things as obesity, Pancreatic Insufficiency, sugar Diabetes, arthritis, bladder stones, skin problems, dental problems, cancer and so on.

Because feeding cereals, particularly rice, is so popular both with the makers of processed foods and with people who devise "home cooked diets" for dogs, I deal with this problem in more detail in Chapter 12.

When You Feed a Commercial Dog Food You Lose Control

Dog foods are like sausages. Mystery bags. This is dangerous! You have very little idea of, or control over what your dog is being fed.

The label might say it contains meat and meat by-products. What does that mean ? It could mean lots of meat, or more likely lots of by-products. Which by-products ? They could be liver and hearts. They could also be feathers and feet ! How would you know. You have lost control.

Look at the protein levels. Is that level good or bad ? How would you know ? Is it good quality protein ? Is it easily digested protein ? How would you know ? You have lost control.

Actually it is usually safe to assume the protein is low in quality and digestibility.

What about the fat. Is there enough ? Is there too much. Is it of the right sort with plenty of essential fatty acids ? You wouldn't know. You have lost control. However, it would be safe to bet that it was of poor quality and low in essential fatty acids.

What about added vitamins. Are there enough ? How would you know ? You wouldn't. You have lost control. Most commercial dog foods contain just enough vitamins to prevent obvious deficiencies, but not nearly enough to cover stressful periods during a dog's life.

Does this food contain toxins ? Such things as lead and pesticide residues. You wouldn't know. You have lost control. In the United States, analyses of dog foods including reputable brands have revealed the presence of these and other poisons as a cause of numerous health problems in dogs. This has occurred on enough occasions to be a cause for concern.

Because our dog foods are manufactured in much the same way and from similar ingredients as the American products, can we believe ours are any different ? You have lost control.

Dog Foods are Made to Match a Scientific Formula

That sounds pretty impressive doesn't it ! Unfortunately it isn't. This method of fixing the nutrients a dog food delivers to your dog is full of problems..... for your dog !

Most dog owners are persuaded that the only way to be sure their dog is getting everything it needs in a nutritional sense, is to feed it a "complete" dog food. One that has a label which implies that the product has every thing a dog needs.

The question is, are these foods nutritionally complete ?

In a recent analysis of pet foods in Australia, it was found that some had less vitamin A than the very minimum levels expected of them. Several had excessive levels. Many dog foods, because of their high calcium levels produce deficencies of other minerals such as zinc and copper.

An obvious problem is that we do not yet know the whole story about nutrition. Much research has and is being done to find out what a dog needs for perfect health. Unfortunately the research is not complete. This means that nutrients about which pet food companies do not have good information could easily be missing from their products.

By law, a dog food which claims to be nutritionally complete only needs to contain certain minimum levels of each nutrient. This is the level which prevents the appearance of obvious deficiency symptoms. The foods are not required by law to contain optimum or best levels of each nutrient. The law does not require that nutrient levels be kept below a safe maximum.

As a result most processed dog foods contain insufficient vitamins for stressful periods in a dog's life such as growth, pregnancy, hard work, surgery, change of home etc..

Most also contain excesses of protein, phosphorus, calcium, magnesium, and sodium. The excess calcium can result in stunting, bloat, zinc deficiencies and bone deformities. Excess protein can result in kidney disease, excess sodium can cause heart disease, excess magnesium causing bladder stones etc..

A lifetime of deficiencies and excesses results in an old age choc-a-bloc with failing organs such as the heart, liver and kidneys.

Apart from the effect of excesses such as calcium causing problems during growth, most of these problems are slow and insidious, and rarely if ever, by the time they have developed, linked to their true cause - that innocent looking commercial dog food.

Although a pet food may meet it's legal obligations if submitted for analysis, that says nothing about the suitability of that product as food which will promote the health of your dog.

It is possible to produce a pet food based on shoe leather, sump oil, coal and water which if analysed will be found to meet the legal requirements necessary for it to be sold as pet food. Unfortunately, there are dog foods around which are not a whole lot better than such a product. This brings us to the next problem with dog foods.

Most Dog Foods are Not Tested Properly

The fact that a dog food can be analysed and found to contain a given set of nutrients says absolutely nothing about whether it will keep your dog healthy, and yet, that analysis is all that the law requires of dog foods.

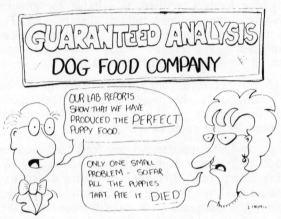

The law does not require that a dog food should be tested by being fed to dogs, despite the fact that such tests are the only valid way to properly assess a dog food. I do not know of a single dog food on the market in Australia that has been tested by actually feeding it to dogs. The tests I refer to are ones designed to find out if it can adequately support growth, reproduction, health, and longevity.

If such a product existed and the results were up to or better than standard, you can be sure the companies involved would sprout those facts far and wide. Their advertisements would tell us all about it!

Instead, we are given advertising campaigns which are often misleading.

For example, because a product is able to be carved does not mean it has the ability to keep your dog healthy.

I have known breeders who were used in advertising campaigns for dog foods. Their dogs had never eaten the products being endorsed.

Not only that, if breeders recommend a product that is a good reason not to use it. All the breeders I have known, keep the things that work for them an absolute and total secret. Their strategy is to pass out poor advice to all and sundry in order to keep ahead of everybody else !

Independent tests carried out in the United States on seven of the leading dog foods advertised as suitable for growing dogs, showed that only two of them fulfilled that promise. The worst two products of the seven resulted in stunted sick puppies, and these were the leading brands. These were foods specifically designed to fill the needs of growing pups !

Although the pet food companies in Australia do not carry out such feeding trials, the people who buy their products do. Often over the lifetime of a dog. I have been observing the results of those feeding trials for years.

I have yet to find a commercial dog food that produces really healthy pups, or promotes dental health, or allows bitches to produce healthy litters, year after year, or allows a dog to become old and remain healthy. They all fail miserably. They look particularly poor when compared to a properly formulated diet based on the raw foods that dogs eat in their natural state.

All Processed Dog Foods are Cooked

This turns out to be a major reason that dog foods fail so miserably. As you read in Chapter 2, when food is cooked it turns into a product for which your dog is not actually designed. The cooking process removes nutrients such as vitamins, enzymes and anti-oxidants and it changes nutrients into unsuitable forms.

The fats, the proteins, the carbohydrates, that is, all the major nutrients in the food are changed. The greater the changes, the more indigestible that food becomes. Also, the more the body regards such molecules as foreign.

These foreign chemicals can result in allergic reactions. The result can be skin problems, bowel problems, even auto-immune diseases like arthritis, and worse than that, many of them are carcinogenic or cancer forming.

In other words, modern cooked and processed foods, not only lack many protective nutrients [vitamins, enzymes and anti-oxi-

dants], but also are full of dangerous chemicals which actively promote cancer and other degenerative diseases.

Dog Foods Have Low Vitamin Levels

The minimum levels of vitamins the law requires in dog foods are much less than the amounts required to promote optimum health in dogs. This is particularly so during times of increased needs such as stress, sickness, growth, pregnancy and lactation.

● Let me give a few examples.

Low vitamin A contributes to skin problems, reproductive problems, immune system problems, growth problems and eye problems. This is unlikely with canned products containing liver and/or kidney. However, vitamin A levels in dry dog foods can be dangerously low.

There is no vitamin C in dog foods. The reason for this is that dogs are capable of manufacturing vitamin C in their liver. However, numerous trials have demonstrated the benefits from added vitamin C during periods of stress. Dogs fed processed dog foods with no fresh foods will suffer a deficiency, particularly during growth, pregnancy and lactation.

Vitamin E plays a major role in preventing ageing and deterioration. Most dog foods have insufficient, resulting in dogs which age rapidly and develop degenerative diseases much earlier than they should.

Dogs that eat only commercial dog food will receive insufficient B complex during periods of stress. This results in nervy dogs that lack energy.

These are only a few examples. I constantly observe amazing improvements in health when dogs are sensibly supplemented with vitamins.

The point to remember about the vitamins in dog foods, is that poor quality products are likely to have major deficiencies. The reputable brands are unlikely to have huge deficiencies. What they are likely to have is marginal deficiencies. Deficiencies which will not cause classical deficiency diseases, but will seriously undermine health during any stressful period. For more information on vitamin supplementation, please refer to Chapter 5.

Dog Foods are Low in Natural and Added Anti-oxidants

Anti-oxidants are nutrients that help prevent degeneration in both foods and living tissues. They are found in abundance together with other anti-ageing and anti-degeneration factors in all fresh foods.

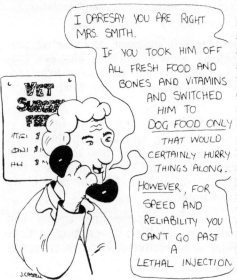

Cooking and processing foods destroys almost all the naturally occuring anti-oxidants and anti-ageing factors. That is why, unless commercial dog foods have extra added, they contain very low levels. This results, particularly in dry dog foods, in the fats going rancid. Dogs eating rancid fats develop poor immune systems resulting in infectious disease, and eventually cancer. Other problems that can result include skin problems and reproductive problems.

Many of these anti-ageing factors are only now being discovered, others are well known vitamins and minerals, for example the vitamins A, C, and E, and the minerals selenium and zinc.

Vitamin E's main function in your dog's body is to act as an anti-oxidant or anti-degeneration factor. Dog foods rarely contain sufficient for it to function adequately in this role.

Processed dog foods do not contain the important anti-oxidant, vitamin C. Although dogs are capable of producing their own vitamin C, when fed processed dog foods, they make much less vitamin C than dogs fed a properly balanced, raw, wholefood diet. The net effect is very low levels of this anti-oxidant available to dogs fed processed dog foods.

Vitamin A has vital anti-oxidant properties. It is present at barely adequate levels in dry dog foods, and some canned products.

Selenium is an essential part of your dog's natural anti-oxidant anti-ageing mechanism. Dog food companies are required to guarantee it's presence in their products. However, we always recommend extra in the form of brewer's yeast or tablets, because it's availability in dog food is in question. Excessive calcium and excessive phosphorus compounds called phytates bind many minerals, including selenium, making it unavailable.

Brewer's yeast is high in other anti-oxidants, the B vitamins, which is yet another excellent reason for adding brewer's yeast to your dog's diet.

This lack of anti-oxidants and other similar nutrients in cooked and processed dog foods is a major reason why modern dogs suffer badly from infectious disease, have problems reproducing, and suffer the whole range of organ breakdown diseases such as cancer, kidney failure, heart disease, arthritis, sugar Diabetes and so on.

Processed Dog Food is Lacking in Food Enzymes

Processed dog foods have no food enzymes. They are destroyed by heat. Food enzymes are a major component of an animals anti-ageing, anti-degeneration mechanism. Food enzymes are known to resist digestion and enter the blood stream. From here they function in a number of ways to reduce ageing and deterioration throughout the body.

They help prevent and possibly reverse the effects of a destructive process called cross-linking. This occurs in all tissues including the skin, the blood vessels, liver, heart etc.. Cross-linking causes deterioration and reduction in function of all parts of the body. It is part of the ageing process.

Enzymes help prevent and even reverse some aspects of joint disease or arthritis. That is part of the reason fresh fruits and vegetables are important in alleviating arthritis in older dogs.

Food enzymes also help digestion. They have a sparing effect on the pancreas. Their absence plays a major role in the development of such problems as Pancreatitis and Pancreatic Insufficiency, both of which are caused in part by cooked "enzymeless" foods.

Processed Foods are Low in Essential Fatty Acids

This has already been mentioned in connection with dry dog foods. Essential fatty acids are nutrients commonly found in plant oils, and chicken and pork fat. They are like vitamins in that they are essential for the proper functioning of your dog's body. A deficiency will cause your dog to develop a range of diseases, including problems with growth, reproduction and the most awful skin diseases.

Beef fat is commonly used in commercial dog food. It is cheap and available. Unfortunately it only has about three percent essential fatty acids. That is why dogs fed commercial dog foods, particularly dry dog foods, often suffer the effects of an essential fatty acid deficiency.

A lack of essential fatty acids is the basic cause of what I call the "dry dog food syndrome".

Dogs with this problem develop a range of symptoms. These include skin probems which often involve the ears, and feet, but eventually the whole body.

These dogs smell, they itch, their skin is often moist, rancid and infected. It flakes and crusts. Their hair coat is sparse, broken, dry and lustreless. Their demeanour is always unhappy. This problem is common, common, common ! It is the basic skin disease, upon which ninety to ninety five percent of all skin diseases are based.

It sells a fortune in drugs and medications year after year, particularly during the warmer months when these pitiful skin conditions become rampant.

Unless the cause of "dry dog food syndrome" is addressed by changing the diet, recovery is rare, despite hundreds of dollars spent on cortisone injections and tablets, antibiotics, creams, washes, etc. etc..

This syndrome can take months or years to develop. If a dog is being fed other foods, the form it takes may be shaped by those foods, as will the time taken to develop and the severity of the condition. Individuals and breeds show varying levels of sensitivity to these nutritional atrocities.

In summary, the low levels of essential fatty acids in commercial dog foods, particularly the dry dog foods are a major cause of much ill health and misery in modern dogs. The presence of essential fatty acids in bone based diets makes a major contribution to the excellent health enjoyed by dogs fed that way.

Most Commercial Dog Foods Contain Nutrient Excesses

Dog foods are not required by law to provide OPTIMUM or ideal levels of nutrients. So long as that product contains each nutrient in excess of a legal minimum, there is no limit to the amount it can contain. Excesses of any nutrient are not illegal.

This is one of the most insidious and dangerous aspects of commercial dog foods. Vets and dog owners often worry about nutrient deficiencies, but we rarely worry about nutrient excesses. Unfortunately, too much of a nutrient can be just as harmful as too little, and it is the nutrient excesses in most of the presently available dog foods which cause a large number of the major health problems seen in dogs today.

- After cancer, kidney disease and heart disease are the leading causes of death in the modern artificially fed dog. The excesses of salt, phosphorus and protein commonly present in dog foods, when consumed over a lifetime are a major cause of both kidney and heart disease. In other words, commercial dog foods are known to be a direct cause of the leading killer diseases in older dogs !

The excessive levels of calcium produce growth problems, particularly skeletal problems, reproductive problems, immune system problems and skin problems.

An obvious question arises.

Why Provide Excesses of Nutrients ?

Why would a dog food company increase costs this way ? There are a number of reasons.

- Firstly, pet food companies may not be aware that excesses of nutrients can be just as harmful as deficiencies.
- Secondly, although it is harmful, it is not illegal.
- Thirdly, most Australian pet foods are multi-purpose.

They are designed to feed all dogs including those which are pregnant, growing and lactating. This means other dogs which are adult and desexed, automatically receive excessive levels of many nutrients for their whole lives.

- Fourthly, pet foods are made from a wide variety of raw ingredients with different nutrient contents.

So that the final product always meets the minimum legal requirements, it is safer for the manufacturer to add more rather than less.

- Finally, many of the raw materials, waste products of the human food industry, are excessive in certain nutrients.

For example, with lots of boneless chicken being produced for humans, there are masses of chicken carcases available. These carcases consist largely of bones. Once cooked and ground into bone meal, and added to pet food, they result in excessive calcium being present in that food. This situation is very common.

The irony is, that raw chicken carcases are an excellent type of raw meaty bone. They keep our dogs wonderfully healthy.

This is a perfect example of the dangers of food processing.

The Problem with Protein Excess in Commercial Dog Foods

Most dog foods contain more protein than is necessary for the average pet dog.

When a dog is fed too much protein, there is a waste product left over which has to be eliminated. This makes the kidneys work harder. Over a long period of time this damages the kidneys.

That means *most pet animals eating commercial dog food are quietly having their kidneys destroyed.* A possible exception is where dogs are eating poor quality dry foods deficient in protein. However, the generally low quality of these products hardly makes them something to recommend.

The kidney damaging effects of commercial dog foods are not well known. This is because the damage takes so long to occur that it is rarely attributed to the true cause. The food.

This problem is very much associated with pet foods being "complete foods". There is reason to believe that those same levels of protein, fed on an intermittent basis, as is the case with natural foods, do not cause the same damage. The problem seems to be the constantly high levels of protein.

The problem with Phosphorus Excess in Commercial Dog Foods

Dog foods in both the United States and in Australia contain between 5 and 9 times more phosphorus than our dogs require. This has a damaging effect on a number of organs, particularly the kidneys.

If a dog takes in excessive phosphorus, most of it is removed by the kidneys. This does not cause a problem.

However, if the kidneys are damaged, for example by a diet containing too much protein, or by bacteria from badly infected teeth, those kidneys cannot get rid of that phosphorus. The result is that both phosphorus and calcium are deposited in the kidney. This causes further damage. That damage results in even more phophorus and calcium left in the kidneys. A vicious cycle of progressive kidney damage is set in motion.

Because commercial dog food usually contains excessive protein and phosphorus it is the perfect kidney damaging food. Excessive protein starts the damage, and excessive protein and phosphorus carries it on.

Once that kidney damage begins, other soft tissues become involved. The lining of the stomach, the heart and the lungs receive deposits of calcium and phosphorus. As a result they begin to function less and less effciently.

However, when phosphorus intake is restricted to normal levels, even with damaged kidneys, no further damage to the kidneys occurs.

Dog foods should contain only the minimum amount of phosphorus. Just enough to meet the animal's requirements. That is, about 0.2%.

As I mentioned, they are currently running at levels of 5 to 9 times that amount. This is very damaging to the health of our dogs.

The Problem with Salt Excess in Commercial Dog Foods

Dog foods in Australia contain anywhere from 10 to 20 times more salt than our dogs require. Is that bad for our dogs ? Unfortunately, yes it is. That excessive intake of salt, or to be more precise, that excessive sodium intake increases the blood pressure in some animals just as it does in some people. Our dogs become hypertensive. This increase in blood pressure causes the same problems in dogs that it does in people. KIDNEY and HEART disease. In fact, studies have shown that this increased salt consumption will still cause kidney damage without an increase in blood pressure.

The Problem with Calcium Excess in Commercial Dog Foods

Most of the commercial dog foods in Australia not only contain excessive levels of salt phosphorus and protein, they are also grossly excessive in the amount of calcium they contain.

Our dog foods contain anywhere from 3 to 11 times more calcium than is necessary to meet the ordinary dog's requirements, with the dry foods on average being more excessive than the canned dog foods.

Is that excessive calcium harmful ? In a word ..YES. This will surprise a lot of people. Many people are absolutely frantic and relentless in their search for calcium supplements for growing puppies. What they do not realise is that practically all our dog foods contain way too much calcium. That extra calcium is already harming our dogs, including our growing pups. There is certainly no need to add more !

When a dog takes in excessive calcium, the excess is not absorbed. It passes out in the faeces. However, while in the gut that excessive calcium binds to other minerals making them unavailable to be absorbed by the dog. They pass straight through with the faeces. That means a dog food may be shown by analysis to have adequate quantities of minerals, and yet the animal eating that product will obtain insufficient to meet it's requirements.

Minerals commonly affected in this way include phosphorus, iron copper and zinc.

Phosphorus will not be a problem because most dog foods already have way too much.

However, it can occur with iron, copper and zinc, and quite possibly with trace minerals such as selenium and chromium.

Doubtless many of our breeding problems relate in part to marginal iron and copper deficiencies resulting in anaemia. This anaemia is a direct result of a combination of excessively high calcium in commercial dog foods together with calcium supplementation by eager owners.

However, by far the most common deficiency occurring as a result of excessive calcium intake, is a zinc deficiency. This zinc deficiency can result in skin problems, growth problems, reproductive problems and reduced resistance to disease.

As you read on, keep in mind that what I am describing is very, very common in a wide range of dogs eating many different commercial dog foods. They are usually the dry dog foods but they can be the ones in a can. They can also be poorly formulated home made diets. The problems are always made worse when the owner ALSO supplements that diet with extra calcium, as is so common.

The first group of dogs most commonly affected by a calcium-induced zinc deficiency are the pups, and one of the first effects you will see in pups is a dramatic decrease in their growth rate, particularly pups of the arctic circle breeds.

- Many skin problems in both adult and juvenile dogs are due in part to a calcium-induced zinc deficiency. The following usually takes a few months to develop.

The first thing you might notice is a generalised thinning of the hair coat and a loss of colouration. This loss of hair colouration may also be due to a calcium-induced copper deficiency. A closer inspection of the skin reveals a dry, flaky dermatitis, which can progress to thickened, crusting, flaky skin.

Other effects caused by a zinc deficiency include delays in wound healing, loss of body protein, decreased nervous system function, decreased function of the thyroid gland, decreased immunity and resistance to infectious diseases, bone abnormalities in growing pups, and testicular degeneration in growing pups. That is a pretty awful list if you stop and think about it.

- Unfortunately there is more !

Excess calcium also predisposes to BLOAT in dogs. When a dog, particularly one of the large deep-chested breeds takes in excessive calcium, that dog responds by increasing it's production of a hormone called gastrin. One of the effects of this increased gastrin secretion is that both ends of the stomach [the intake end and the exit end] thicken, making it difficult for gases to escape. As a result, it becomes difficult for these dogs to either pass gases further down their digestive tract, or to belch them out, thus making it very easy to develop bloat when the conditions are right.

Another problem now being attributed to the excessive levels of calcium in commercial dog food is dental tartar and all the problems which stem from that !

The bottom line to all of this is that feeding processed dog foods with their excessive levels of calcium is not a terribly great idea, and adding extra calcium to these diets is an even worse idea !

The Problem of "Complete and Balanced" ... the "Stew" Mentality

One of the problems with home cooked food, but more especially commercially produced dog food is that it attempts to combine all the nutrients a dog needs to stay healthy in the one food.... all cooked up together.

This is an unusual approach to feeding anything, and causes innumerable health problems.

With the passage of time, this particular problem will be found to sit alongside cooking as one of the major reasons processed foods are so damaging to the health of dogs.

The most significant problem with this method of feeding, particularly when it is combined with cooking, is that it allows nutrients in the food to interact with one another. This interaction between nutrients prevents many nutrients from being available for your dog. The most common example is the interaction I have just described. The one between the excessive levels of calcium in processed foods and other minerals such as zinc, chromium, selenium, iron etc. These nutrients become unavailable and the health of your dog suffers.

Another related problem is the presence of those very same minerals in such a food. Their presence, particularly when added as a supplement and combined with heat, inactivates a number of vitamins, particularly members of the B complex.

These types of problems do not occur when a wild dog or a modern dog fed in a primitive way receives it's nutrition. The food is not cooked and is not "complete and balanced". This promotes health because it minimises the chances of one type of nutrient interfering with other nutrients as I have just described.

The second type of problem involves the mixing together of starchy foods and protein rich foods in the same meal.

Some of the early work done by scientists trying to understand digestion involved dogs. During the 1930's an American doctor, examined this earlier work in dogs and as a result advocated the separation of starch rich meals and protein rich meals in his human patients in an attempt to improve digestion and therefore health.

The results were astounding. Just this simple change in the way food was presented lead to seemingly miraculous improvements to health. For example, it promoted normal weight where previously there had been either under or over weight. This principle is in accord with what happens in nature.

In other words, it seems highly likely that this food separation and food combining effect may be part of the reason that dogs fed in a more natural manner are much healthier. Conversely, it is a major reason that dogs which are fed processed foods, the supposedly "complete and balanced" ones, are so unhealthy.

Chapter 6 is devoted to food separation and combination.

Processed Foods may Contain Chemical Toxins

We have no way of knowing the long term effects on our dogs, of the continual consumption of toxic chemicals potentially present in dog foods. Particularly with regards to the production of tumours or cancer. Unfortunately, the presence of toxic chemicals in commercial dog food is a distinct possibility because of the origins of the raw ingredients.

Processed foods are made from three types of ingredients. Firstly there are the by-products of the human food processing industry. These include plant wastes such as the outer coats of grains and other wastes from the milling industry. On the animal side, the wastes include such things as hearts, spleens, lungs, guts, livers and bones etc..

The second type of ingredient used to make dog foods are the sheep, cattle, pigs, chooks etc. passed as not fit for human consumption. That is, the four D's, the dead, the dying, the diseased and the disabled animals at the slaughter houses.

The third type, mainly plant products, are the grains and vegetables purchased or grown specially for manufacturing processed dog food.

It is possible for all of these to contain hazardous toxins.

Unfortunately there is no way of knowing whether the particular batch of processed foods being fed to your dog contains chemical toxins or not. To test each batch of dog food would be incredibly costly, and yet that would be the only way to ensure a trouble free product.

For example, the four D's, the animals not fit for human consumption. Why were they not fit ? Many of our farm animals suffer with the toxins and poisons from modern industry. A common example are the cattle which graze by the roadside all their lives. They suffer from chronic lead poisoning. In America, cases of lead posioning in dogs have been attributed to such cattle ending up in dog foods. It is believed by some vets that much of the modern epilepsy seen in dogs can be attributed to such toxins, particularly chronic undetected lead poisoning. Lead poisoning in dogs has also been attributed to solder used to seal the cans, leaking into the canned food.

The outer coats of grains which make up a large proportion of many dog foods should be treated with suspicion. They harbour the residues of a host of chemicals which include such things as insecticides and herbicides and fungicides etc. etc.. Many dogs, like humans are quite susceptible to even minute traces of such chemicals.

- This possibility of toxins in dog foods is another valid reason for dog owners having more control over what their dog eats rather than leaving it in the hands of a dog food company. A company with no particular interest in the long term health of household pets.

All this talk of toxins in dog food may sound alarming. However, it is a bit like death due to snake bite and death on the road. There are far more deaths due to road accidents than snake bites, but we tend to fear snakes more than we do cars. In this case, most of the other problems I have outlined are far more important to the health of your dog than the presence or otherwise of toxic chemicals in dog foods.

However, we do live in a very polluted world, so that the presence of such toxins in a lot of food, both canine and human is a very real possibility, and a probable cause of much chronic poor health. For this reason it should not be ignored, and this is another valid reason to be wary of commercial dog food.

Some Dog Foods are Worse than Others

This is important. Many people think all dog foods are much the same. In fact they are not, some are much worse than others.

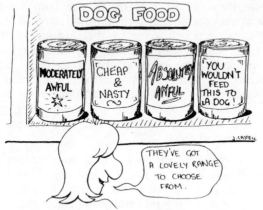

The problem is, knowing which are the better ones. Which are the best of a bad lot. In the long run, only time and experimentation [feeding the stuff to your dog] will tell you. However, price is a guide. You mostly get what you pay for.

In that respect, there are three groups into which we can lump the different brands of dog foods.

Firstly there are the "no name" or generic brands. These are usually the cheapest.

Secondly there are the middle of the range "popular" brands. The ones that advertise on national television at mealtime. They have a middle of the range price.

Thirdly there are the "vet only" brands. That is, dog food, available only from your vet on prescription. These are expensive, and are used to treat specific disease conditions such as heart failure, obesity, kidney failure etc., particularly in the elderly dog.

Let me repeat that in general, price is a fair indicator of quality.

No Name Plain Label Generic Pet Foods

These "el-cheapo" pet foods, have no particular brand names. They are produced from the cheapest, poorest quality materials, with little or no quality control. They are guaranteed to have low digestibility, low nutritional value and excesses or deficiencies of any or all of the nutrients. There is no guarantee that the product will always be the same. One week the product may be poor, but the next time you buy it, it may be terrible.

In the long term they become very expensive. More has to be fed to meet an animal's needs and the poor health they result in means added expense for the owner, and misery for the animal.

Popular Brands of Dog Foods

These are the brands which advertise at dog shows, on TV at mealtime, and in the national canine journals.

These are the brands most people buy. People believe what they are told. They believe that these foods are the best available.

Such is the power of advertising, dog owners continue to buy these products even when their dogs have numerous health problems. Advertising fools a lot of people in all sorts of ways, not the least of these being sales of dog food.

Prescription Brands

Prescription brands are the most expensive brands of pet foods available.

This is because no matter what the cost, the same raw ingredients must always be used. No substitutions are allowed as happens with "normal" dog food.

Another reason is because they are mostly imported. However, that is beginning to change as local manufacturers realise the potential for profit in this market.

Another cost factor is the amount of research required to enable the production of these products.

Finally, anything which can be tagged "medical" or "prescription" attracts a higher price tag.

These dog foods are designed to "treat" animals with one or more of the degenerative diseases, including obesity. They treat diseases produced in the main by a lifetime spent eating other processed dog food. They achieve their effects by strictly controlling the levels of energy and certain nutrients such as minerals, protein, salt, phosphorus etc. which they deliver to the "patient".

Each has a very strict formulation. They are called prescription diets because the correct one must be selected for a particular disease condition. This involves a vet correctly diagnosing which degenerative disease is involved. It is also because in some cases their use in a normal animal may cause problems.

Kidney disease is a good example.

Most kidney disease in modern dogs is the result of a lifetime spent eating commercial dog foods. Those foods damage the kidneys with their excesses of phosphorus, salt and protein and also because they produce dental problems. The dental problems result in a diseased mouth acting as a focus of infection which eventually affects the kidneys. Once the infection is cleared up with dentistry and antibiotics, the kidney degeneration is held in check by one of these prescription diets which has limited levels of phosphorus salt and protein.

Dogs which spend a lifetime eating bones and other more natural foods, rarely if ever require the services of these expensive processed prescription diets.

"Boutique" Brands of Dog Foods

Because of the marginal to poor results seen with so many of the "been-around-a-long-time" commercial dog foods, there are now lots of "new" dog food companies springing up all over the place. Some small, some quite large, including brands selling worldwide.

Unfortunately, although these products may contain better quality ingredients, and therefore be somewhat better than your average commercial dog food, in my experience they are not all that much better. Not so as you would recommend them anyway.

They are still cooked. They still have various nutrient excesses and deficiencies, and in fact, are probably even more excessive in protein than "ordinary" dog foods. Not only that, they still cause massive dental problems, and most important of all, the results they produce are still poor.

The results can be an improvement over those obtained with the better known or popular brands, but they are not all that encouraging compared to a properly formulated diet based on whole raw foods.

The bottom line with feeding is that it is the results that count!

A FINAL WORD ABOUT COMMERCIAL DOG FOODS

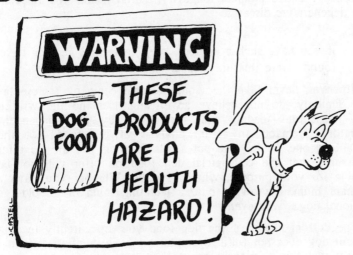

So far as commercial dog foods go, the best you can say of them is that they are useful as a stand by when other foods are not available. The circumstance I am alluding to is where the only other alternative was death by starvation.

My general advice regarding most of the dog foods currently available is that if you run out of food for your dog, it would be far better to give your dog a healthy twelve or twenty four hour fast, rather than feed it commercial dog food.

Commercial dog foods should never be regarded as complete and adequate diets. Always assume that they will contain both nutrient excesses and deficiencies and will not produce optimum health in your dog.

● There are only two exceptions to that rule.

The first is where you have scientific data which has demonstrated a product's suitability when being fed for the purpose for which you require it. That data will include dental health, and lifetime studies must have been carried out.

The second exception is where you are feeding your dog on a commercial dog food, and that dog is in tip top health, and you know that that particular food has been demonstrated in controlled trials to promote longevity, dental health and freedom from degenerative diseases.

● If you have such a product, keep on feeding it. You have found a rare treasure indeed.

However, never take the word of some company representative. Similarly, do not believe advertising. Demand the written proof of actual feeding trials performed by an independent laboratory. Demand an actual analysis of the food, not the guaranteed one. If they are not available, then you are far safer to assume that the commercial dog food on offer will not be suitable for your purpose, whatever it be. Whether you have a pregnant mum, a growing pup, a lactating mum or an old-age pensioner dog.... whatever.

The bottom line is, if the dog food you are curently feeding to your dog does not fulfill the criteria I have mentioned, then I suggest you think seriously about changing your dog to a more health-promoting diet based on raw meaty bones. If you are still not sure, keep reading. The next chapter looks at the problems inherent in, and caused by, home cooked and home produced dog food.

- 4 -

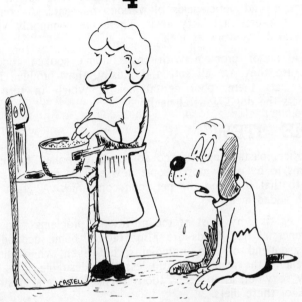

Common Problems with Home Produced Dog Foods

Unfortunately, many of the people who realise that commercially produced dog food does not produce worthwhile results, devise and cook up something which is in essence not very different from the processed food they were worried about. As a consequence, the results in terms of the health of their dog is not a whole lot better.

Not uncommonly, home produced dog food suffers from both excesses and deficiencies of various nutrients. A common deficiency is essential fatty acids. There are commonly vitamin and mineral deficiencies as well.

A major problem with these home cooked foods is that because they are all soft and mushy, they produce in the dog that eats them, poor dental health, which in turn adversely affects the dog's general health.

THE "STEW"

Rice, pasta, veggies and some meat cooked up into a stew seems to be what most people devise. This recipe is pretty similar to that followed the pet food companies. A grain based diet with added meat.

That is why most of the nutritional problems associated with commercial dog foods are also true of home cooked stews. It does depend on the ingredients, but even when these appear excellent, the results are still less than desirable. This is particularly so when grain based foods such as rice and pasta form the bulk of these diets.

The main problem apart from the cereal base and no bones is that stews, in common with most home produced dog food are cooked. This means they will be lacking in many vitamins, food enzymes, and natural anti-oxidants.

A related problem, is that because stews are a cooked all-in-together type of food, there is the possibility of interactions between nutrients, making some of those nutrients unavailable. There will be none of the benefits to health of food separation.

On the plus side, the product will not be a mystery bag. The cook can ensure that only good quality ingredients are used with no added flavourings or colourings, and it is unlikely to contain toxic materials. The mix would probably contain a whole lot more vegetables than are used in the commercial product.

However, in the final analysis, my experience with these stews, is that they do not produce good results in terms of the health, reproductive ability and longevity of dogs. The results are sometimes better than seen in the the dog fed on commercial dog foods, but not good enough for me to recommend this method of feeding.

A COMMON ERROR - THE SINGLE ITEM DIET

One of the most common feeding errors made by dog owners attempting to formulate a diet for their dog, is to feed only a single food item.

Sometimes lots of different foods are offered, but the dog selects the one he or she wants. This is particularly so in the case of small dogs. Usually, larger dogs are "general stomachs" and will eat anything offered. What follows are some of the single item diets that people feed their dogs, or which the dog selects.

Feeding all or Mostly Organ Meats

This is not terribly common in dogs. It mostly happens with cats. However, I have seen it done.

One dog fed that way was on a steady diet of liver, kidney, tongue, heart, brains and a bit of steak. For a couple of months he looked fantastic, because he had been switched from a commercial dog food diet to this all organ meat diet. It was obvious at first that his new diet was giving him much that had been missing from his previous diet of dry dog food. For a while his body was back in balance.

However, as time went by, his body became unbalanced in other directions. He became very lethargic, developed skin problems, arthritis, and started vomiting after nearly every meal.

He had developed a form of hepatitis, and had a very high cholesterol reading. He required months on a low protein, mostly vegetable diet to regain a semblance of normality.

This diet of organ meat was excessive for calories, protein, phosphorus, vitamin A and was very deficient in calcium. It probably had other imbalances, but these were the obvious ones.

In short, don't do it !

Of course feeding organ meat to your dog in small amounts as part of a balanced diet is great. Very good for your dog. It only becomes a problem when it is the only food item fed.

Feeding Mostly Fish

Once again, this is more likely to be a problem with cats. It is mostly a problem when only the flesh is fed. Do not feed your dog on an all fish diet, particularly if the flesh is the only thing you feed. There will be problems. Raw fish flesh can contain an enzyme which destroys vitamin B1, and if the fish is exceptionally oily, your dog may develop a vitamin E deficiency as well. Oily fats go rancid easily. In the process, they use up vitamin E.

Of course fish flesh as a small part of a balanced food programme for your dog is fine. Just don't feed it as the only food fed.

A number of people I have spoken to over the years have fed their dog on lots of whole fish... raw ... including the head, the guts and the bones. Their dogs did not have problems. Presumably, because when the whole fish was fed, any missing nutrients, e.g. B vitamins and vitamin E were supplied by the brain and the eyes and the intestines of the fish.

Feeding Your Dog an All Meat Diet

- This is a very common feeding error.

Lots of people feed their dog on a meat only diet as a simple and hopefully more healthy alternative to any of the commercial dog foods. Sometimes cooked, sometimes raw. It also happens a lot with little dogs owned by the elderly. Little dogs usually train their older owners to feed them single food items, and that single food item is commonly meat.

Over the years I have seen many dogs, fed on mostly cooked meat, develop problems such as arthritis, eczema, kidney and heart disease and very commonly cancer.

It is common for the dog food companies to use this feeding error, the all meat diet, because of the problems it causes, as the reason dog owners should use their product. Dogs switched from an all meat diet to a commercial dog food will do exceptionally well - for a while, and then gradually decline in health as the problems inherent in the commercial product take over.

So what is wrong with an all meat diet ? Surely that is what wild dogs eat ? Yes they do, plus a whole lot more besides !

Meat fed by itself is a totally unbalanced diet for a dog.

First and foremost, meat only contains a minute fraction, about 4 %, of a dog's calcium requirements. This is disasterous when puppies are fed this way, and no good for adult dogs in the long term either.

That meat only diet is also deficient in iodine, copper, vitamin A, vitamin E and vitamin D. On top of that, an all meat diet is excessive in both protein and phosphorus.

Feeding an all meat diet to a growing pup will totally ruin that pup in about a month. It will take longer to see problems in an older dog.

A lot of people try to correct the deficiencies in an all meat diet by adding calcium. A common figure is two teaspoons of calcium carbonate per kg of meat. That may correct the calcium deficiency, but it does nothing for those other deficiencies and excesses I have outlined.

In short, the all meat diet is a disasterous way to feed any dog, but is particularly bad for a growing puppy. Don't do it !

However, that is not to say that you should not feed your dog or your growing puppy meat. Of course you should. You just have to feed it as part of a balanced diet. Not as the only thing fed.

Feeding Table Scraps Only as Dog Food

Almost everybody who has asked their vet what they should feed their dog has had the experience of being told not to feed table scraps. They are told that if they MUST feed their dogs table scraps, under no circumstances should those table scraps make up more than 25 % of the diet. The remainder absolutely must be provided from balanced good quality commercial dog food.

Why do vets say that ? After all, for most of their evolutionary history as an associate of man, dogs have lived on the scraps from man's dinner table.

The reason your vet advises you not to feed table scraps is

because he or she knows that in many cases, feeding table scraps as the major part of the diet can result in a diet that is highly unbalanced.

Vets have noticed that when table scraps are fed to dogs, they mostly consist of two food groups ..... fat and carbohydrates. That is, they are mostly meat trimmings, which are nearly all fat, and vegetables, which are carbohydrates. Sometimes there will be a lot of gravy, which of course is fat and carbohydrate also.

We know that if that was all the dog ate, or that was what made up the bulk of the dog's diet, that dog would soon be showing signs of gross nutrient deficiencies.

Such a diet is almost totally lacking in protein, unless some of the meat is included, and it is also completely lacking in minerals, particularly calcium. It is probably also deficient in a number of vitamins. In short, it is a recipe for disaster.

A diet, that is low in protein and minerals would rapidly cause problems in a growing pup, and would eventually cause problems in an adult dog.

A major problem seen in adult dogs fed this sort of diet is obesity. This is because such table scraps, consisting as they do of loads of fat, carbohydrates and water, are very palatable. A dog eating these all the time would become very obese.

Part of this problem is that many dogs become addicted to such food..... refusing to eat anything else. In fact, as they become more obese, and more unhealthy due to such an un-balanced diet, they even more stubbornly refuse all other food.

Once again, table scraps as part of a diet based on raw meaty bones are fine for your dog. This is the way dogs have eaten for centuries. However, as the only food fed over a long period of time, they are usually not a healthy balanced way to feed a dog.

For more information on feeding table scraps to your dog, please refer to Chapter 15.

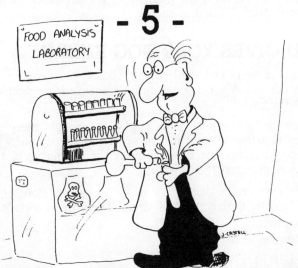

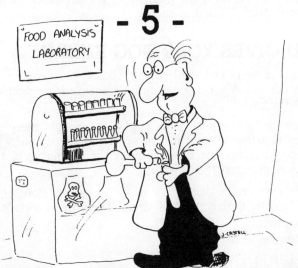

- 5 -

Food - What is in It ?

The function of this chapter is twofold. Firstly, to give a brief review of the major nutrients in food, including proteins, fats, carbohydrates, minerals and vitamins etc., and secondly to develop a list of commonly available food items which can be used to feed your dog.

The chapter does not provide an in-depth course in basic nutrition. The aim is to provide a mini-crash-course in nutrition for those who have no training in this area, and to serve as a memory jolt for those who have forgotten.

As we work our way through the basic nutrients, various food items will crop up as supplying each of them. That means by the end of the chapter there will be a list of food items from which to choose when organising your dog's diet.

Not only that, you will be able to make those choices based on a knowledge of the nutrients each food supplies.

That is why, even if you do have sound basic nutritional knowledge, I suggest you at least skim this chapter.

I shall start off with the most important substance or thing to be found in food. That is..... energy.

FOOD GIVES YOUR DOG ENERGY

Energy is fuel. The stuff which allows your dog to run all day and not tire. Your dog can get it's energy from proteins, fats and carbohydrates.

If you do not supply your dog with enough energy foods, your dog will lose weight. If you supply too many energy foods - your dog will become obese. This is the beginning of the end for many dogs - and their owners !

There are certain times in a dog's life when more energy is needed. Usually during times of stress. These times include:

- Growth
- Reproduction
- Activity
- Cold periods
- Hot periods.

The reason a dog needs more energy during hot periods is because it's cooling mechanism - panting, uses an enormous amount of energy.

During any of these periods of increased stress, you have to supply either more food or food which is more energy rich. If you want a more energy rich food, the obvious choice is a fat rich food. Fat is the most energy rich nutrient available, having more than twice as much energy as a similar weight of protein or carbohydrate.

A common mistake made by a lot of dog owners is to con- tinue feeding their adult dog like a puppy. That is, they feed it as if it were still growing. Disaster! All that unneeded extra energy has to go somewhere. The end result is a fat, immovable lump of a dog, doomed to a host of problems.

So do think about how much energy your dog requires. If your adult dog is getting too much energy in it's food, he or she will get fat. If your dog is not getting enough, weight loss will occur.

This is the basis of deciding how much food to give your dog. That is, you look at it and/or weigh it, then feed it accordingly, to keep it at a constant healthy weight.

A Quick Run Through The Energy Nutrients - starting with -

Carbohydrates - Mostly Not Needed

Carbohydrates are the foods produced by plants. These include, the soluble carbohydrates or simple sugars as found in fruit, honey, commercial dog foods, sugar cane, the sugar bowl on the table etc..

They also include the insoluble or complex carbohydrates known as starches, as found in grains and vegetables such as the potato, pumpkin etc., and also found in commercial dog foods.

- There is another type of carbohydrate. That is, the indigestible but highly important substance called fibre. Fibre has a unique role to play in the health of your dog, particularly the soluble fibres found in vegetables.

In an evolutionary sense, carbohydrates are important to man as a source of energy, but not to dogs. Unfortunately, modern dogs are forced to eat a lot of starch when they eat commercial dog food or homemade grain-based diets. Most commercial dog foods have loads of starch because they have grains as their main ingredient.

Many commercial dog foods also have heaps of simple sugars, another food which dogs have never eaten in abundance. These are added to act as a preservative and to make the food more appealing or appetising. This helps sell the product. People buy the food which their dog will eat !

Commercial dog foods and many homemade diets contain varying amounts of fibre, also coming mostly from grains. This type of insoluble fibre, like sugars and starches, has not figured prominently in the dog's diet before the advent of commercial dog foods.

As you might be gathering, starch, simple sugars, and insoluble fibres, are not foods a dog's body is designed to handle in large amounts for long periods. Yet that is precisely what we ask our modern dog to do when we feed commercial dog foods and some home cooked diets.

Modern man feeds these products to dogs from the standpoint of convenience and least cost. Dogs are not fed this way because it is best for them. In fact, not only does the dog not require starch and sugar to stay alive and be healthy, there is mounting evidence suggesting that modern starch and sugar-rich dog foods are hostile to their health.

There is only one time a dog actually requires carbohydrates. Research has shown that pregnant bitches need some carbohydrates if they are to produce a healthy litter. Even here, because the research was done with processed foods, such conclusions are suspect in terms of a dog on it's natural diet.

Although wild dogs are not programmed to eat masses of grains rich in starch, they regularly eat carbohydrate-type foods. They eat the intestinal contents of their prey. This food is rich in carbohydrates, such as a variety of sugars, small amounts of starch, and lots of soluble and insoluble fibre.

Our modern dogs should be getting their carbohydrate in a similar manner and balance. The best way to do this is to feed dogs lots of fresh, whole, raw vegetables. Vegetables contain lots of soluble and insoluble fibre, some starch and simple sugars.

If this is to be successful, the vegetables must be properly prepared. That is, they should mimic the intestinal contents of a dog's prey. They must be completely crushed. In that way the nutrients in the vegetables become available for digestion, and therefore useful to the dog. More than that, they promote health, so that their consumption is to be encouraged. Refer to chapter 10 for details.

On the other hand, grains, and products such as pasta should be limited severely. Particularly rice, wheat and corn. More of that shortly.

Fat - Your Dog Needs It !

This is the most energy-rich nutrient available for your dog. Pet dogs which do not have to work hard for their food like wild dogs, do not require a lot. Excess causes obesity leading to disease and possibly death.

However, your dog needs some fat in it's diet. Fat, especially animal fat, makes food more palatable. Fat provides insulation, including the insulation of the body's wiring system - the nerves. It provides physical protection and padding. It enables the absorption of the fat-soluble vitamins, A, D, E and K. It is an essential part of the structure of every cell membrane in your dog's body. Fats give rise to hormone like substances called prostaglandins. Some fats contain essential fatty acids. Your dog's body cannot manufacture them. They must be supplied in the diet.

Essential Fatty Acids

Essential fatty acids are like vitamins. Without them disease occurs. They are part of every cell membrane in your dog's body. If absent, their place is taken by non-essential fatty acids. This causes disease.

Essential fatty acids are used to produce a group of hormone-like molecules called prostaglandins. Prostaglandins help regulate every aspect of a body's functioning. With a fatty acid deficiency, that regulation goes badly wrong producing disease.

Dogs fed on processed and cooked foods often lack essential fatty acids. This causes those inflamed itchy skin conditions seen daily in veterinary hospitals throughout the western world.

Their lack also causes growth problems in puppies, fertility problems in both sexes and is involved in all the degenerative conditions of old age.

Dogs fed a diet rich in saturated fats such as beef tallow, or monounsaturated fats such as olive or canola oil, are more likely to develop a deficiency of essential fatty acids, than dogs fed a diet rich in chicken fat or lard, or one of the polyunsaturated vegetable oils such as safflower oil, soya bean oil, or corn oil.

Dogs fed a diet rich in polyunsaturated fats will have problems if an antioxidant such as vitamin E is not fed as well. This is because the fat will literally go rancid in the body.

WARNING: do not feed your dog margarine. The fatty acids it contains, although made from plants have been changed to a form foreign to the bodies of most mammals. There is very good evidence that the extensive use of these products contributes to an increased incidence of cancer.

There are Two Families of Essential Fatty Acids

Omega 6 Fatty Acids

This group of essential fatty acids are found in the vegetable oils, poultry and pig fat.

Diets which are lacking in these essential nutrients produce skin problems, reproductive problems and growth problems. The diets involved include practically all dry dog foods, most other commercial dog foods, and most home cooked diets based on rice and beef with no oil added.

Commonly available sources of the omega 6 fatty acids, include safflower oil, sunflower oil, soya bean oil, corn oil and cotton seed oil. Safflower oil has one and a half times as much as the other four. Peanut oil has about one third the level of safflower oil, while linseed and olive oil have one fifth and one sixth the amount respectively. Pork fat and chicken fat have about one third the level of safflower oil.

Omega 3 Fatty Acids

The second family of essential fatty acids is known as the omega 3 family. Their lack will cause both nervous and vision problems and learning difficulties in puppies. Male animals require them to be fertile. The most common source is fish and fish oils. Most modern diets also lack sufficient levels of this group of essential fatty acids.

They are available to wild dogs in brains, eyes, raw eggs, faeces and the plant material in the rumen of their prey. Wild dogs eat much more of this group of essential fatty acids than modern dogs fed on processed foods and poorly constructed homemade diets. That is why modern dogs suffer from so many allergic and inflammatory skin problems, arthritis, and other "allergic" conditions

Plant foods rich in the omega 3 group of essential fatty acids include linseed oil - the richest non marine source, followed by rapeseed oil [one fifth the amount, followed by soya bean oil [one seventh the amount], then corn oil and all the other vegetable oils with small amounts.

WARNING: The linseed oil you feed to your dog must be "food standard". Buy it from a health food store. Linseed oil as used to treat timber etc. is totally rancid and therefore poisonous to your dog.

Other plant sources with small but significant amounts of the omega 3 group include oats, mushrooms, baked beans, spinach and bananas.

Animal sources are lamb's liver and rabbit. These have the highest levels, with other meats having small amounts. Surprisingly lean beef has higher levels than lean chicken.

Fish liver oils should not be used as a source of these essential fatty acids because of the danger of overdosing with vitamins A and D.

- If all of this sounds confusing... do not be alarmed. Just include in your dog's diet a broad range of the foods I have mentioned which contain the omega 6 and omega 3 groups of fatty acids. That is, lots of raw, meaty, chicken bones, eggs, brains, lambs liver, rabbit, green leafy vegetables, oats, mushrooms, baked beans, spinach and bananas, together with an appropriate vegetable oil supplement.

Of the oils you might use note that both corn oil and soyabean oil contains a good balance of the omega 6 and the omega 3 family of essential fatty acids.

- ## THE IMPORTANCE OF VITAMIN E

If you are supplementing your dog's diet with oils and fats high in essential fatty acids, you must add vitamin E to the diet to prevent rancidity of these fats in your dog's body.

All oils fed to your dog should be fresh. They are best stored in air-tight containers in the dark. This is to minimise rancidity.

Similarly, it is not wise to take used cooking oil and feed it to your dog. There is a distinct danger of poisoning them with already oxidised [rancid] oils. In this respect, the hard fats are safer.

Proteins - Give Your Dog the Best !

Apart from being a source of energy for your dog, proteins, together with fats form the basic structural material which makes up your dog's body. That is why your dog has to have a lot more protein in it's diet when it is growing, than when it is an adult. When your dog has stopped growing it only needs enough to replace what is lost through wear and tear.

There are two exceptions to that rule. The first exception is when your bitch is pregnant. Then, she needs extra protein to help the pups inside her grow. The second exception is when she is feeding those pups on the milk she produces. At that stage she needs even more protein than when she was pregnant.

Protein also functions in a whole host of ways as that most important molecule called an enzyme. *Enzymes are molecules found in every cell and every part of your dog's body. Their role is to enable the chemical reactions which are the basis of your dog's life, to proceed at the proper pace and in the proper manner.*

Just as fats are made from fatty acids, and there are particular fatty acids which are essential and therefore have to be included in the diet, so it is with proteins. That is, proteins are huge molecules consisting of many thousands of amino acids, some of which are known as essential amino acids. These are the ones your dog's body cannot manufacture. This means it is far more important that our dogs get the correct balance of essential amino acids rather than a given amount of proteins.

For the record, the following amino acids have been designated as essential for the dog. Threonine, valine, methionine, isoleucine, leucine, phenylalanine, histidine, tryptophan and lysine.

Those names are given for information only, please do not let them confuse you.

Protein Quality

Protein quality is governed by two factors. The presence or absence of essential amino acids, and the ability of that particular protein to be digested and absorbed.

Thus a poor quality protein can be deficient in two areas. It can be poor quality because it lacks one or more of the essential amino acids,and it can be poor quality because your dog is unable to digest and absorb it easily.

A common example of a poor quality protein, deficent in both ways is the protein present in a dry dog food or any diet constructed mainly from cereals.

A lot of commercial dog foods contain protein that has low levels of certain essential amino acids and is not easily digested. Manufacturers get around this is by supplying excessively high quantities of this poor quality protein in the product mix.

Another way of thinking about proteins is that they are the main nutrient found in meat and eggs and cheese and milk. That is a great way to think of proteins. When you think of those particular proteins, you are thinking of good quality proteins.

To balance up the protein in cereals, feed a legume food in equal amounts to the cereal food. E.g. - add baked beans.

Better still, switch to a properly formulated diet based on raw meaty bones which have an excellent balance of the essential amino acids.

The Results of a Protein Deficiency

These include a failure to grow or reproduce properly, anaemia, poor hair coat, weak thin muscles, a poorly functioning immune system, bones that do not grow properly, in fact, any part of your dog would be badly made and function poorly. It is common to see this in puppies raised on poor quality dry dog foods or poor quality cereal based homemade diets.

Most modern dogs on commercial dog food suffer a protein excess. I have already spoken about the protein excess problem and pointed out that the problem may lie with constantly high protein diets caused by attempting to make each meal a complete and balanced one. I pointed out that the more natural way to feed a dog is to achieve balance over time. By doing that, many meals will be low in protein giving the dog's kidneys a rest.

So how much protein do dogs require ? If the protein was of first class quality, a growing or lactating dog would do quite well on about 18 % protein. A non reproducing dog would suffer no deficiencies if fed a diet containing 8 % - 10 % good quality protein. The only problem with food containg the lower levels of protein would be reduced palatability.

- Protein of high quality includes the protein from egg, cottage cheese or lean beef etc.
- The protein in most dog foods is derived from poor quality plant protein, so that much higher amounts are required.

That is why most of the commercial dog foods have up to 4 times the amount of protein that dogs actually need. That poses no problem for the lactating dog and the growing dog, but if an adult dog is maintained on that level of protein for it's entire life, given at every meal, as when commercial dog food is fed, it will eventually suffer kidney problems.

There is in fact much controversey on protein levels. As dogs age, they lose the ability to utilise it efficiently so that they actually require more in their diet. However, the vast majority of dogs eating commercial dog food, because of constantly high protein levels throughout life have damaged kidneys. To control that damage requires low protein diets.

- This has resulted in scientists who study ageing and nutritional requirements in dogs recommending that older dogs, particularly those with declining kidney function be fed smaller quantities of better quality protein.

All this research has been done with dogs eating processed foods. My own limited research and extensive observation of dogs fed primitive diets where high protein meals containing high quality proteins have been fed intermittently all a dog's life, suggests that this way of feeding may allow higher protein levels to be fed and not cause kidney problems.

In other words, a more logical approach is to prevent the problem in the first place by copying nature and providing high quality protein for a dog's entire life, but not at every meal.

If your dog's diet is based on a wide variety of raw meaty bones, with those bones and their attached meat making up about 60 % of the diet, you can stop worrying about proteins. Your dog is getting the best !

MINERALS - Bones Make it Simple

A variety of minerals must be supplied in your dog's diet in correct balance and sufficient amounts if he or she is to grow properly and stay healthy, and in the case of breeding dogs, be able to reproduce.

The two needed in greatest abundance are calcium and phosphorus. These are found mainly in bones. They give bones their strength. There are many more minerals such as zinc, magnesium, manganese, iodine, selenium, chromium, iron etc., which your dog requires as an essential part of it's bodys structure and functioning.

Wild dogs relied principally on raw meaty bones as their source of a balanced complement of minerals. Our modern dogs can do no better than follow their example.

Do realise your dog will not, cannot, suffer mineral deficiencies, imbalances or excesses, when raw meaty bones make up the bulk of it's diet. This applies to dogs of all ages, including puppies. And I don't just mean puppies of the smaller breeds. I mean all breeds of puppies, including most definitely the giant breeds.

This is because bones are the storehouse of all the minerals your dog requires in perfect balance, and in the perfect form for optimal absorption with no excesses or deficiencies. Of course this is hardly surprising. It is natural for dogs to eat bones. A dog's body is designed to use bones as it's main source of minerals. This is what dog's bodies have been doing for millions of years.

Feeding dogs in any other way is courting disaster as is testified daily by the problems, including mineral imbalances seen in dogs fed without bones, particularly where calcium supplements are used instead.

Modern dogs fed without bones, suffer a multitude of mineral imbalances. These include:

Calcium Deficient Diets

Dogs fed on home made diets, such as table scraps but no bones, or mostly meat diets suffer from a deficiency of many minerals, but most particularly, they suffer a deficiency of calcium. This used to be a common problem. However, the pendulum has swung the other way. The most common mineral problem suffered by modern dogs is an excess of calcium.

The Excessive Calcium in Commercial Dog Foods

The most overwhelming problem with modern processed foods so far as minerals are concerned is their huge excess of calcium. That excessive calcium produces very poor availability of minerals such as zinc, iron and copper, and many other vital trace minerals including chromium and selenium.

The Excessive Salt in Commercial Dog Food

The second major mineral excess in Commercial dog foods is salt. Most commercial dog foods in Australia contain way too much salt. This is part of the reason many of our dogs suffer hypertension and cardiovascular disease.

The Excessive Phosphorus in Commercial Dog Foods

The third major mineral excess in commercial dog foods is phosphorus. That too causes its share of problems including a large proportion of the old age kidney failures we vets are forced to treat.

Every dog consuming processed dog food, or cooked food as the bulk of it's diet is suffering one or more of these mineral imbalances to a greater or lesser degree.

The Problems of Mineral Suplementation

Supplementing a dog's diet with minerals can be an extremely hazardous affair. In the case of a puppy, the results can be instantly disasterous, with skeletal problems and skin problems and growth problems following rapidly.

In older dogs, the problems can take longer to develop, but it is not uncommon for many arthritic, skin and internal problems to be a direct result of a lifetime mineral imbalance. That is, the result of being fed a commercial dog food or poorly formulated home made diet, or diets which have been indiscriminately supplemented with minerals, particularly calcium.

Another mineral causing increasing concern is zinc. Many people, having heard that zinc is important because a lack of it will cause a myriad of problems, begin supplementing their dog's diet with zinc. The results of a zinc overdose are equally disasterous as any other mineral imbalance, particularly in the growing pup. This can happen with any mineral you might choose to supplement in isolation.

Bones - The Only Logical Way to Supply Your Dog With Minerals

Bones, together with the other dietary elements recommended in this book are in fact the only truly logical way for your dog to get it's correct balance of calcium, phosphorus and other minerals, particularly the growing pup.

The other dietary elements which help bones to supply your dog with it's correct mineral balance include foods such as fresh, green, leafy vegetables, a variety of fresh meats - lamb, beef, chicken, organ meats, dairy products, seafoods, eggs, brewer's yeast, kelp powder or tablets and small amounts of whole grain foods.

By feeding such foods in addition to the raw meaty bones, you are making doubly sure your dog is getting all the minerals needed in perfect balance.

VITAMINS

Please read this section. It is perhaps the most important part of this chapter. Vitamins are crucial to your dog's health, and there is an incredible amount of mis-information regarding vitamins and the modern dog's requirements.

Most modern dogs do NOT need supplementing with minerals, particularly calcium, But often receive them in abundance to the detriment of their health. On the other hand, dogs which do require vitamin supplementation for maximum health, often receive none at all.

First - What are Vitamins .....

There are approximately sixteen organic substances or chemicals recognised by science as vitamins. Chemically, most of them are completely unrelated. However, every one of them is an essential component of the normal chemistry of the body.

Without them, bodily functions do not proceed, and neither, eventually, does life. Most unprocessed raw foods contain one or more of them. If insufficient vitamins are present in an animal's diet, disease is inevitable.

Their common names reflect the order in which they were discovered early this century. Hence vitamin A, B [complex], C, D, E etc.

Vitamins Have a Much Wider Role in Health Than Many Suppose

In Australia, the addition of nutrients to breakfast cereals goes back some thirty or more years. This is because thirty years ago, deficiencies were detected in the Australian population. So it came about that Australian foods could be legally fortified with vitamins A, C and D, thiamin, riboflavin, niacin, and the minerals iron, calcium, phosphorus and iodine.

These laws are being revised, and it is being proposed to no longer allow the addition of calcium, riboflavin, vitamins A and C, and to reduce the amount of iron that can be added.

The argument in favour of these reductions is that by no longer allowing the addition of vitamins and other healthy additives to foods, manufacturers of junk foods will be unable to make unsubstantiated health claims for those foods. Sounds a bit like commercial dog food doesn't it ? You know, unsubstantiated claims based on the presence of certain nutrients. But actually - that is not my point.

The point I am coming to is that leading nutritional scientists are very much in opposition to reducing vitamins in foods, and argue that we humans ought to be consuming more rather than less vitamins. Modern veterinary literature is advocating exactly the same thing.

Until recently, vitamins were thought of as substances whose only function was to prevent deficiency diseases. To do this, only very tiny amounts of each vitamin are required. We now know they have many more functions which require them to be present in the diet at much higher concentrations.

To help you understand this let me introduce you to the concept of .....

The Five Possible Levels of Vitamin Supply

The First Level is the "Not Enough" Level.

This will result in severe deficiency symptoms such as blindness with insufficient vitamin A, or the disease scurvy with not enough vitamin C.

The Second Level is the "Barely Adequate" Level.

This is the level which is sufficient to prevent any signs of the classical deficiency diseases. For example, no scurvy due to a lack of vitamin C. No blindness due to a lack of vitamin A.

If your dog eats one of the better brands of dog food, most

of the vitamins will be at this second level. The barely adequate level. Insufficient vitamins for maximum health.

The Third Level is the "Present in Abundance" Level.

Dogs in the wild usually receive their vitamins at this level. They have access to a wide variety of plant, animal, and mineral materials. These foods contain an abundance of naturally occuring vitamins.

This level sees vitamins present at concentrations many times greater than is necessary to simply stop obvious signs of a classical vitamin deficiency. They could vary from 5 - 100 times the amounts present at the second level.

At this third level, the vitamins act as a buffer against stress.

They promote:
● Health
● Stamina
● Reproductive ability
● Disease resistance
● Longevity.

They allow:
● Hard work
● Pregnancy
● Lactation
● Growth.

They support
● The proper functioning of the immune system.

They help
● The body remove toxic chemicals.

These toxic chemicals are derived from an increasingly polluted environment. These pollutants cause problems during growth and reproduction and hasten many of the degenerative diseases of old age. Vitamins that fight pollution include vitamins A and C.

- The third level allows for individual variation in the amount of vitamins required.

While some dogs may do reasonably well at the second level, others may not function properly until the vitamins are present at this third level.

In other words, for optimum health, our dogs should receive their vitamin supply at this third level. That is, in abundance like their wild ancestors.

The Fourth Level of Vitamin Presence is the "Pharmacologic Level".

Here, massive but non toxic doses of vitamins are given to achieve drug like effects. Hence the name pharmacologic dose. These levels can be used to treat disease problems.

The Fifth Level of Vitamin Presence is the Toxic Level.

For some vitamins, e.g. the B complex group, and vitamin C, it is almost impossible to get to the fifth or toxic level, whereas for other vitamins such as vitamin A and vitamin D, toxic overdose is a distinct possibility.

Modern Dogs Lack Sufficient Vitamins

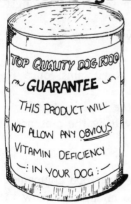

Most modern dogs fed on either commercial dog food or home cooked food receive most of their vitamins at the second or barely adequate level, and in some instances, at the first or not enough level.

This is of major concern because it is a cause of much ill health. Rarely do we see the total absence of any of these vitamins, although very occasionally we do.

More often, what we see is a state of chronic poor health. Nothing major, nothing you can diagnose as a definite disease problem, just a dog that is not as active or as bright or as happy as it could be.

All of these dogs are more prone to infectious disease, to parasites such as fleas and worms. However, what starts out as a series of apparently minor problems eventually progresses to serious disease. Such dogs age early, and they suffer a multitude of degenerative disease problems such as cancer, arthritis, skin diseases, kidney disease, heart disease etc. If the dog is owned by a breeder, it will have problems reproducing.

The question you have to ask yourself is why do these dogs lack sufficient vitamins for top notch health ? In other words, what is wrong with modern foods ?

Why Do Commercial Dog Foods Lack Vitamins ?

There are at least five reasons why commercial dog foods lack vitamins in abundance. Why they have vitamins at the second level only.

- The first reason is because most commercial dog foods are made from a limited number of ingredients.

The commercially fed dog is eating a product containing mostly cooked grain and grain by-products, cooked animal and animal by-products, plus some vitamin and mineral supplements. This is in contrast to the wild dog which scavenges amongst a broad array of food stuffs.

- The second reason is because many vitamins are destroyed by heat.

Even if the food was originally rich in vitamins, once it is processed, many vitamins are lost.

- The third reason is because when the food is mixed together, many vitamins are destroyed by the presence of the mineral supplements.

This effect is made worse by cooking.

- The fourth reason is that when the dog food companies add extra vitamins, they do not add enough to allow the vitamins to be present at that third level of abundance.

They add just enough to get their product to that second level, where in theory there should be no symptoms indicating a vitamin deficiency.

- The fifth reason is that in the case of dry dog foods, the vitamins are quickly lost if the product is not consumed soon after manufacture.

This is made worse by poor conditions of storage, including heat, light, moisture and being left open to the air.

Why Home Cooked Foods Lack Vitamins

The reasons are much the same as for commercially produced products. That is, they are often made from a limited number of ingredients, many of the vitamins are destroyed by heat, and with the home cooked product, usually no vitamins are added back in to the product at all.

The net result is that modern dogs are left with no protection, no buffer to shield against stress.

I regularly witness improvements in the health of dogs supplemented with extra vitamins. This is particularly so during critical periods such as growth, reproduction and old age. I see these improvements with dogs eating commercial dog foods, home cooked foods, and even dogs on so called natural diets following vitamin supplementation.

The Vitamins Themselves

I now want to take you for a quick tour of the vitamins themselves. I want you to get an idea of what they do in your dog's body, the sorts of foods that they are found in, and the levels at which they may be safely and usefully supplemented.

It is not important to memorise or even fully understand this information. Instead, I want you to get a "feel" for the vitamins. To become aware of how important an adequate supply of them is to your dog' health. To understand that their role goes way beyond the mere prevention of deficiency symptoms. To realise

the wide ranging health promoting roles they have to play in the
normal internal workings of your dog's body, when they are supplied in adequate amounts.

Types of Vitamins

There are two broad groups of vitamins. The so called water
soluble vitamins and the fat soluble vitamins.

The water soluble vitamins are vitamin C, and the B complex
group. The fat soluble vitamins include vitamins A, D, E, and K.

The B Complex Group of Vitamins

These are ALL water soluble vitamins. They are the ones the
body is supposedly unable to store. However, that is not true.
The body stores all of them to a geater or lesser degree. It can
take weeks or months for a deficiency to occur when they are
lacking in the diet.

The reason I make this point is because many people are
under the impression that if these are not supplied on a daily
basis, ill health will result. That is of course nonsense. It is part
of the myth which says each meal you feed an animal has to be
totally baalnced. Let me emphasise and reinforce the importance
of achieving a balanced diet over time - weeks, not at each
meal.

- On the other hand if you give your dog a huge amount
  of any of these vitamins, there is no problem. One
  hundred times the recommended dose of any of them is
  quite safe. Whatever your dog's body does not need and
  cannot store will be piddled out with absolutely no harm
  done. On the contrary, you will be making sure that your
  dog is receiving adequate amounts of these most essential
  nutrients.

The B Complex Group - Their Functions

The B complex group are vital for energy production. They
take part in all phases of the conversion of fats, carbohydrates
and proteins into energy. Without adequate B vitamins, no
energy is produced for your dog's normal bodily functions, for

activity, for growth etc.. Insufficient amounts of B vitamins produces a weary, lacking-in- energy, growing-obese dog.

They are essential for the proper functioning, development
and maintenance of the nervous system, including the production
of neuro-transmitters. ["signals" within the nervous system.] They
have a generally calming effect.

Without adequate levels of the B vitamins there is poor development, reduced functioning and inadequate maintenance of the
immune system. They are involved in such things as the production of antibodies and the proper development of the thymus
gland which is the master gland of immunity.

Many of them function as anti-oxidants. That is, they are responsible for preventing ageing and degeneration of tissues, including the elimination of dangerous molecules produced inside
and outside the body, called free radicals. They are involved in
preventing the degenerative process called cross-linking.

The B vitamins are involved in dealing with stress, including
the manufacture of bodily cortisone - the anti-stress hormone,
and the production of vitamin C, a major anti-stress vitamin.

The B vitamins are involved in all phases of growth, reproduction and repair of body tissues. They are vital for all stages
of blood production, and are necessary for the health of the
entire body including the production and maintenance of healthy
skin, hair and sweat glands, the maintenance of internal organs,
and for the health of sense organs like the eye and tongue.

They are involved in, and essential for, all aspects of the
body's functioning including such diverse activities as production
of fatty acids, controlling hunger, controlling blood cholesterol
and triglyceride levels, stabilising blood sugar, assisting in the
normal functioning of the thyroid and adrenal glands etc..

- Let me emphasise once again that it is not necessary for
  you to understand or remember all of those functions.
  Just realise that all those bodily functions are vital for the
  normal functioning of your dog. In other words, The B
  complex vitamins in adequate amounts are of absolute
  importance to the health of your dog at every stage and
  in every phase of it's life.

What Foods Contain These Essential B Vitamins ?

Modern foods rich in members of the B complex include brewer's yeast, whole grains including brown rice and oat flakes, wheat germ, wheat bran, wholemeal bread, muscle meat, the organ meats - heart, brain, liver and kidney, eggs, especially the yolk, raw chicken, cheese, yoghurt, milk, fatty fish, green leafy vegetables, root vegetables, peas and potatoes, molasses, dried fruits and fresh fruit and vegetables.

Of the above, only brewer's yeast and liver contain close to the whole range of B vitamins. In other words, to ensure your dog receives plenty of these essential nutrients, feed most of those common foods to your dog - for all of it's life.

As I will emphasise continually, it is not necessary for each meal to contain all the vitamins. In other words, feed all of those foods over weeks or even months. That way balance will occur over that period. This is normal and healthy for all animals.

I also want you to realise how much more available the B complex group of vitamins are in fresh whole foods, and that the more food is tampered with by processing, particularly cooking, and the more foods are mixed together during cooking, the greater the chance of one or some or all of these vitamins becoming deficient to a greater or lesser degree.

What you will see when dogs are not fed properly, and where one or more of the B complex are in short supply, will be a multitude of vague health problems which to date have never been assigned any particular cause. The sort of vague problems with no particular name, seen daily in vet surgeon's offices. The problems that occur as forerunners to one or more of the more serious and more developed and therefore more diagnosable disease conditions.

The good news is, all these vague problems are totally and easily preventable when your dog is fed a properly balanced diet based on raw meaty bones, and including plenty of vitamin-rich foods as mentioned above.

If in any doubt at all about the adequacy of the diet you are feeding your dog with respect to the B complex group of vitamins, supplement that diet with a balanced mix of all of them.

This can only be beneficial to your dog. These can be obtained from a chemist, a health food store, a supermarket or from your vet.

- B vitamin supplements are best given with food,
  otherwise they can be irritating for your dog's stomach
  lining.

Just remember, it is almost impossible to give your dog an excessive amount of the B complex group of vitamins. As a rough guide, anything suitable for a child will be suitable for a dog.

To emphasise how safe they are, realise that it would be quite safe to give a toy poodle a human adult dose of B vitamins. Not only would it be safe, you would be ensuring that they were being supplied at that third or super abundant or health promoting level. In other words you will be increasing the possibility of owning a healthy dog !

Vitamin C - Your Dog Needs Extra !

Vitamin C is a water soluble vitamin. Like the B group of vitamins, vitamin C is often thought of as a vitamin the body is unable to store. However, as with the B complex that is not true. Your dog's body does store vitamin C. In other words, just as it is not essential to supply the B vitamins on a daily basis, so it is with vitamin C.

However, as with the B complex group, large amounts of vitamin C on a daily basis are not toxic. What your dog's body does not need and cannot store will be piddled out with absolutely no harm done. On the contrary, you will be making sure that your dog is receiving a super abundant supply of this most essential and non toxic vitamin.

Ask most modern "experts" about dogs and vitamin C, and you will be told that dogs do not need vitamin C in their diet because they are capable of manufacturing it. That is half true. Yes they are capable of manufacturing some of their own vitamin C, but for maximum health they should also be fed food rich in vitamin C, or at least be given vitamin C as a supplement.

Wild dogs receive much more vitamin C in their diet than domestic dogs. It is present in the fresh organ meat and in the stomach contents of the animals they prey upon. The berries and fruits they constantly scavenge are rich in vitamin C. Because they eat foods rich in vitamins and other nutrients, they also make more vitamin C than the modern unhealthy dog fed on cooked and processed foods.

That is why for all round good health, our dogs must receive far more vitamin C than most of them can presently manufacture or is supplied in their commercial dog food or cooked food diet. Commercial dog food has none, and home cooked food often has very little.

In other words, modern dogs miss out in two ways. Firstly they receive a diet with little or no vitamin C in it, and secondly, because of the general poor quality of their diet, they are unable to make large amounts of it, particularly during stressful periods when more is required.

Vitamin C is the Anti-Stress Vitamin

Stress is the major factor causing an increased need for this vitamin. During periods of stress, your dog's requirements of vitamin C rise sharply.

Stress Situations Which Respond to Extra Vitamin C.

TOXIC INSULTS Vitamin C is a major weapon in the fight against poisons. It helps eliminate the poisonous heavy metals from the body. Things like arsenic and lead, all too common in our modern world.

DISEASE STRESS Megadoses of vitamin C are of benefit in resisting and fighting various infectious diseases, including viral diseases.

SURGICAL OR TRAUMATIC STRESS Vitamin C concentration increases in the tissues which surround a healing wound. This is because it is actively involved in the healing process.

TRANSPORTATION STRESS This includes moving house, going to dog shows, or to a vet, or a boarding kennel.

REPRODUCTIVE STRESS Extra vitamin C prior to, during and after mating will promote your dog's immune system and boost it's general resistance to disease problems. It will help to reduce or eliminate infertility and birth problems. Vitamin C during pregnancy aids in promoting an easy, rapid, stress-free birth.

THE STRESS OF LACTATION When she is feeding pups, a female dog is under tremendous stress. Extra vitamin C ensures both her continuing health and the health of the puppies.

WEANING This is a time of great stress, particularly when it is combined with finding a new home. Extra vitamin C is definitely indicated at this time.

GROWTH STRESS Rapid growth is a stress which responds to additional vitamin C. Vitamin C is essential for the production of the protein collagen which is the major structural component of all living tissue. Bone problems caused by rapid growth often respond to supplementary vitamin C. Of course the growth should be slowed as well !

PHYSICAL EXERCISE Vitamin C helps fight fatigue, and ensures rapid repair of tissues worn and damaged during heavy exercise.

OLD AGE AND DEGENERATION Ageing is a process which is slowed down remarkably by the addition of vitamin C to the diet.

WEATHER STRESS Sudden heat, cold, rain, or being hit with strong winds etc. causes stress. Dogs faced with any of these should receive extra vitamin C.

How Much Vitamin C is Needed ?

Like the B complex group, vitamin C is completely non toxic. Sensible supplementation of this vitamin can only be of benefit. As I have already mentioned, any not needed is passed out of the body - in both the urine and the feces.

Large amounts of vitamin C will cause diarrhoea in the dog. This is not dangerous. Reduce the dose and the diarrhoea stops.

• Use this method for determining the maximum dose of vitamin C. This is called the bowel tolerance method for determining the dose of vitamin C.

If you follow my recommendations of feeding fresh whole foods including plenty of green vegetables, the normal daily requirements of vitamin C will be always available both from the diet and because your dog will manufacture plenty of it.

However, as with the B vitamins, there is no harm in supplementing your dog's diet with extra. Particularly during periods of stress. On the contrary, you can only benefit the health and longevity of your dog by adding extra vitamin C to the diet.

Of course there will always be individual animals which will require constant dosing with vitamin C. This is also true where dogs live in pretty contaminated environments, such as big cities, near busy roads, next to factories and so on.

Recommended Doses of Vitamin C

A daily supplement of vitamin C at the rate of about 50 to 100 mg per kg will do no harm and can only ensure the continuing good health of your dog. As your dog's stress levels increase, so you should increase the amount of vitamin C given.

SLIGHT STRESS - 100 mg/kg

MODERATE STRESS - 200 mg/kg.

HEAVY STRESS - 300 mg/kg.

VERY HEAVY STRESS - 350 mg/kg.

As you increase the dose rate of Vitamin C, it is important to divide the daily dose. That is, do not give the whole dose all at once. In other words, for slight stress, divide into two doses, with moderate stress, divide into four doses, and for heavy to very heavy stress, divide the total dose into about six doses. You may use the "Bowel Tolerance" method as described at the top of this page for determining the maximum desirable dose of vitamin C to give. As the stress passes, gradually reduce the dose back to the non stressed dose rates.

Use the non stressed dose rate for the dog eating a diet based on raw meaty bones etc.. That is, a primitive or natural diet containing plenty of vitamin C. For the dog eating a predominantly commercial dog food diet, or a mostly cooked diet, the minimum amount recommended as a supplement is the level for moderate stress, that is, between 100 and 200 mg/kg daily.

● In severe stress, you may give your dog the top level of vitamin C or even more, up to the point it causes diarrhoea.

Forms of Vitamin C

Vitamin C exists in several different forms. Vitamin C itself is ascorbic acid. The two common salts of vitamin C are sodium ascorbate and calcium ascorbate. There is another form of vitamin C called ester C.

Mostly it does not matter which form you use. However there are some exceptions. For example, it would be better to give a dog with arthritis either calcium ascorbate or ester C or perhaps sodium ascorbate rather than ascorbic acid.

You would not give sodium ascorbate to a dog with heart problems because of the presence of sodium. In a young dog with hip dysplasia due to calcium excess, you would not give calcium ascorbate.

The Fat Soluble Vitamins

The fat soluble vitamins include vitamins A, D, E and K. These vitamins have much wider roles to play in the health of our dogs than many people realise. With the possible exception of vitamin D, they are all anti-oxidant or anti-ageing type nutrients.

However, unlike the water soluble vitamins which are almost completely non toxic, the fat soluble vitamins require a little more care. They are much more readily stored in your dog's body, and particularly in the case of vitamins A and D, there is the potential for toxicity if they are supplied at grossly excessive levels.

This problem of potential toxicity has scared many people away from supplementing their dog's diet with fat soluble viamins. Half truths are always dangerous. Sensible supplementation with all of these vitamins at the appropriate dose and at the appropriate time has the potential to be immensely beneficial to most modern dogs.

Vitamin A or Retinol

Vitamin A is a fat soluble vitamin with anti-oxidant or anti-ageing properties. It affects and is required by every part of your dog's body and practically every process in it.

It is essential for normal vision, the proper functioning of the immune system, the maintenance of all mucous membranes, skin health, normal functioning of the adrenal glands and hence stress resistance, all stages of reproduction in both sexes and for normal growth including bone growth.

The addition of this vitamin to the diet of dogs with numerous health problems has proved to be highly beneficial.

Problems are more likely to appear when dry dog foods are being fed. Dry dog foods are notoriously low in vitamin A, particularly if they are not fresh or have been stored badly.

Minimum Levels of Vitamin A Required by Your Dog

Quantities of vitamin A are usually expressed as international units. One international unit of vitamin A is equal to 0.3 ug of retinol.. which is another name for vitamin A.

Dogs being fed a typical middle-of-the-range popular sort of commercial dog food, receive approximately 50 to 100 iu of vitamin A per kg of body weight per day. This means that a 10 kg [22 lb] dog receives approximately 500 to 1000 iu of vitamin A per day, while a 50 kg dog would be receiving 2,500 to 5,000 iu per day.

These amounts are at the second level of vitamin intake. The just adequate level.

Safe Supplementation with Vitamin A

A safe supplement would be 100 to 200 iu of vitamin A per kg per day. That means a 10 kg [22 lb] dog would be given an extra 1000 to 2000 iu per day, while a 50 kg [110 lb] dog would receive between 5000 and 10 000 iu of extra vitamin A per day.

The only time you do not need to supplement is where you are feeding vitamin A rich food such as liver on a regular basis, say once or twice a week. In that case, your dog is probably receiving sufficient vitamin A. Another possible situation where you may need to be careful would be where a canned dog food was being fed which advertised itself as being rich in liver.

In my experience, by adding vitamin A between 5 and 10 times the commercial dog food rate, no problems are encountered with toxicity, and the results in terms of improved health, improved reproduction etc. etc. are dramatic. In this case you are adding vitamin A at the rate of 250 to 500 iu per kg of dog per day. This is the third level of supplementation.

This means a 10 kg dog would be receiving between 2,500 and 5000 iu of vitamin A per day. A 50 kg dog would receive betweeen 10,000 and 20, 000 iu of vitamin A per day.

For periods of 1 to 2 months, for an average dog, such levels are totally safe. Another way to safely supplement at this level is to supplement at this rate for a month, then during the following month give no extra vitamin A, then in the third month supplement again etc..

Situations Where Additional Vitamin A Should Not Be Added

- Severe kidney or liver disease.
- Where a diet is already rich in vitamin A, for example, a diet containing a lot of liver.
- The rare occasion where an individual cannot tolerate the higher levels.

I have not come across such a dog yet, but it is theoretically possible. The only way you can discover such an individual is when signs of toxicity develop. These are listed below. Fortunately it usually only takes a few days to a few weeks for the signs to be reversed.

Authorities agree that generally safe levels for dogs are 4 - 10 times the currently recommended levels, but that these levels can quite safely be exceeded for short periods of time.

Most of the harmful effects have been obtained by feeding over 100 times the daily requirements for many months.

Signs of Vitamin A Toxicity

The signs of toxicity include skeletal malformations, spontaneous fractures, cartilage loss, internal haemorrhage, increased blood clotting time, loss of appetite, slow growth, loss of weight, skin thickening, suppressed keratinisation, reduced red blood cell count, enteritis, conjunctivitis, congenital abnormalities, and problems with the liver and kidney such as degenerative atrophy, fatty infiltration and decreased function.

The Dog's Natural Sources of Vitamin A

The richest sources of vitamin A are fish oils. Vitamin A will also be found in milk fat, egg yolk, and liver. These are all rated as rich sources of vitamin A.... but it DOES depend on the diets the animals they came from were being fed !

Most people rely on supplements such as cod liver oil or more commonly synthetic vitamin A in capsules.

Provitamin A or Beta Carotene is another source, particularly where large quantities of green vegetable material is being eaten. Wild dogs eat plenty of this, and so should your dog. Your dog's intestines convert Carotene into vitamin A.

All green parts of plants are rich in Carotene. The degree of green gives you a rough idea of the carotene content. Carrots, corn, sweet potatoes [the yellow ones], pumpkin, squash and green leafy vegetables are all a good source. All of these are highly recommended as part of your dog's balanced diet.

Vitamin E - the Age Fighter !

Your dog's body is continually attacked by molecules it produces called free radicals. If this is not stopped, it results in ageing and associated degenerative diseases, such as cancer, strokes, arthritis etc. Free radicals are commonly formed when fat in your dog's tissues becomes rancid.

- To survive these attacks by free radicals, your dog relies heavily on vitamin E. Vitamin E, in this it's major role is called an "anti-oxidant". In fact vitamin E is one of the principal anti-oxidant or anti-degeneration vitamins.

Because of it's role as an anti-oxidant, vitamin E plays a major role in retarding the ageing process, treating heart disease, preventing blood clots and therefore strokes in older dogs, disease resistance, healthy reproduction and in protecting against the toxic effects of heavy metals. It is also important in energy production in cells, and in the production of vitamin C.

How Much Vitamin E do Dogs Need ?

This depends very much on the diet. That is, if the diet includes unsaturated oils such as corn oil, cod liver oil, sunflower oil, linseed oil etc the need for vitamin E can increase up to five times. This need is even greater if they are going rancid at the time of ingestion.

Because vitamin E is destroyed when it prevents fats from going rancid, feeding a dog lots of cod liver oil, or any other oil high in polyunsaturated fatty acids and low in vitamin E, will eventually result in a vitamin E deficiency and subsequent tissue degeneration.

The stress of infection increases the need for vitamin E, particularly if polyunsaturated fatty acids are being fed.

A 25 kg dog requires 1 to 5 mg of vitamin E are daily. This is the amount required to bring the vitamin E supply to the second or barely adequate level of intake. However, at least five to ten times more are required when the diet contains lots of polyunsaturated fatty acids, particularly fish oils. This is because most plant oils do contain some vitamin E, while fish oils have none.

- A safe abundant supplementary dose for a dog would be from 10 to 20 mg per kg. That is, for a 25 kg dog, 250 to 500 mg per day.

Natural Sources of Vitamin E

Vitamin E is found in green plants. The vegetable oils have the highest levels of vitamin E, with wheat germ oil having the most, then cottonseed oil, safflower oil, soya bean, peanut etc.

Eggs, whole grains, the germ of grains, liver, legumes and of course all other green plants are all good sources.

Most animal by products contain small amounts but not a lot. Milk is a variable source. Butter is good. Eggs, particularly the yolks are usually a good source, depending on the diet of the hen.

Most animals will benefit from extra vitamin E !

Toxic Effects of Vitamin E

There are virtually no known side effects caused by massive doses of vitamin E. One exception is high blood pressure. Sudden large doses cause a further temporary rise in blood pressure. Older dogs with impaired hearts may have high blood pressure. They will benefit from extra vitamin E, so increase it slowly. That is, give low doses to start with, working up gradually to the required dose. This is best done in conjunction with your vet.

- A dog with rat bait poisoning should not be given high doses of vitamin E. Do not give iron supplements with vitamin E, they have the effect of cancelling each other out.

Vitamin D

Vitamin D is the sunshine vitamin. Your dog can get all it needs by spending 15 minutes in direct sunshine daily.

Inside dogs need it in their diet. E.g. from cod liver oil. Sunlight which has come through a window pane does not produce vitamin D in your dog. Clouds, mist smoke and air pollution all block the production of vitamin D.

What does Vitamin D do for Dogs ?

Vitamin D ensures strong bones containing plenty of calcium. It makes sure the calcium needs of the rest of the body are met. It does this by controlling the absorption of calcium and phosphorus from the intestines and their deposition and withdrawal from the bones, together with regulating their loss or retention via the kidneys.

Requirements

- A young and healthy dog on a well balanced diet based on raw meaty bones receiving plenty of sunlight will not need additional vitamin D.

Dietary Sources of Vitamin D

- Fish liver oils are the best source of vitamin D. It it is also found in salt water fish such as herring, salmon, sardines etc.. Opening a can of sardines occasionally for your dog is a great idea. Milk and butter do not contain much, nor do most meats.

- Egg yolks can be a good source of this vitamin if the diet of the hen contained plenty, or if it had spent plenty of time in the sun. On that basis you would have to think seriously about buying free range eggs !

Supplementing Your Dog's Diet with Excessive Vitamin D

After vitamin A, vitamin D is the vitamin most likely to be toxic if you give too much. Excess vitamin D causes excessively high levels of blood calcium.

The result is widespread deposits of calcium throughout the body, disrupting normal bodily functions.

Upper Safe Levels of Vitamin D

These are 4 to 10 times the currently recommended levels for periods in excess of 60 days, and up to 100 times the currently recommended levels for periods of less than 60 days.

The currently recommended levels are 22 iu per kg of dog daily for a growing pup. This means that a level of 100 iu per kg per day would be a good safe but abundant level. Hence a 5 kg puppy could receive 500 iu per day, or 3500 iu per week.

Cod liver oil has about 10 000 iu of vitamin D per 100 gm [approximately one hundred ml], this means that 35 ml would supply a 5 kg puppy's weekly requirements, which works out at about one teaspoonful daily. However, that dose would be excessive for vitamin A, so only give one teaspoon per week of cod liver oil.

Effects of a Vitamin D Deficiency

Rickets, or weak bendy bones will occur in young pups if they do not get adequate vitamin D. This problem is made worse by insufficient calcium in the diet. The first sign will be poor growth, loss of weight, and reduced appetite. Next you see problems with the bones, including curved, bent, easily fractured bones plus enlarged hock and knee joints. That typical bandy-legged appearance.

The adult counterpart of this disease is Osteomalacia. With this disease, the bones gradually get thinner and weaker. It usually takes years to develop. The main symptoms are muscular weakness and bone pain. Eventually there are bone fractures.

The practical circumstances where this would occur are in old dogs that have lost the ability to manufacture vitamin D, dogs that are on a poor diet such as dried or canned dog food or an all meat diet, and dogs that are rarely in the sun.

- Dogs kept constantly on a healthy diet based on raw meaty bones, spending plenty of time in the sun will not develop this problem.

Vitamin K

This is known as the antihaemorrhagic vitamin. It ensures your dog's blood clots following cuts and scratches. It helps the liver produce various blood clotting factors.

It is also one of the many anti-oxidant or anti-ageing nutrients, Recent research suggests it also has an essential role to play in reproduction and growth, particularly bone growth, and in the production of healthy skin.

Vitamin K is made by bacteria living in the large intestine of your dog and also in most other animals. This means that dogs which eat faeces usually get plenty. It can also be absorbed directly from the bowel, meaning that for most healthy dogs a deficiency is unlikely.

Dietary sources of vitamin K include green leafy plants, and on the animal side, fresh liver and fish. It is particularly rich in fresh dark green vegetables such as the outer leaves of lettuce, cauliflower, broccoli, brussel sprouts and spinach.

Dogs taking lots of antibiotics, particularly sulphonamides, may have reduced bowel production of vitamin K.

Vitamin K is another great reason to feed a wide variety of foods including plenty of green leafy vegetables to dogs of all ages, but particularly to reproducing and growing dogs. For the older dog, requiring food with anti-ageing properties, vitamin K rich foods are also a great idea.

Vitamin K is basically non toxic, particularly the natural forms. However, the synthetic forms can be toxic with the toxic dose being in excess of 100 times the recommenced dose. The recommended oral dose is .05 to 1.0 mg per kg of body weight.

It should be noted that vitamin K is the antidote of choice when your dog eats warfarin-based rat baits. These baits have an anti-vitamin K effect.

Supplementing Your Dog's Diet with Vitamins

I put forward the following thought for those of you who are still sceptical about adding vitamins to your dog's food.

There is an equation used in determining public health policy for humans.. it reads as follows... "If there is a fifty percent chance of doing some good, and a one hundred percent chance of doing no harm, then that justfies some action."

- I hope by now that you are convinced that the addition of vitamin supplements to your dog's food if done properly, has an almost 100 % chance of doing no harm and has much more than a 50 % chance of doing some good.

WATER - WORTH SOME THOUGHT

I don't know if you have thought about it, however, we and our dogs, in fact any land mammal can only go for a few minutes without air, a few days without water, but many weeks without food. In other words, next to a plentiful supply of fresh air, the most important and essential nutrient your dog needs constantly is water.

Unfortunately, tap water is one of the ways modern man is polluting himself and his animals. The major problem is that the chemicals used to clean our drinking water, by destroying the bacteria are now thought to be reacting with natural substances found in the water to produce chemicals which may cause long term genetic damage and possibly cancer.

A major problem for Australia is that we do not have a uniform set of rules governing the protection of our nation's water. The rules vary between States and between regions within states. Another major problem is that many of the so called safe levels of faecal and chemical contamination are based on levels set for Europe, which was heavily contaminated before the rules were set. What this has meant in practical terms, is that the authorities in Australia have given private and government bodies a licence to pollute our waterways, and our drinking water.

This I give you as food for thought. Obviously we all need water. Our dogs are no exception. It is quite possible for the water your pet drinks to cause it some problems. Probably not from the bacterial content, our dogs, particularly our healthy dogs will deal with that a lot better than us. The main danger is the masses of chemicals to be found in the water.

Water treated by water filters may be a very good idea for chronically ill pets, or pets having reproductive problems or growth problems. If the water where you live is such that you need to do that for yourself, then it will also benefit your pet.

The provision of truly clean water as another aid in producing a healthy dog is worthwhile thinking about.

ANTI-OXIDANTS AND ANTI-AGEING FACTORS

Natural whole foods, that is raw, unprocessed foods contain a lot of natural molecules which fight the processes of degeneration and ageing. That is, they contain anti-oxidants and other anti-ageing factors. Most of these molecules have not been identified. Unfortunately Many of these elusive molecules are destroyed by heat and other food processing activities.

This means, that for your dog to attain maximum health, you either have to add these substances back into the food, or alternatively, feed the raw primitive foods which have not lost them... e.g. lots of fresh fruit and vegetables, together with raw meaty bones.

The good news is that apart from those as yet largely unidentified compounds, many vitamins, the ones we have already discussed have strong anti-ageing/anti-oxidant properties. This is particularly so in the case of vitamins A, C and E.

- In other words, it is not a bad idea to feed the primitive diet AND add vitamin supplements as a way of giving your dog a diet high in anti-ageing/anti-degeneration nutrients !

The subject of these nutrients and the ageing process is discussed more fully in the last chapter.

THE LIST OF FOODS SUITABLE FOR FEEDING NORMAL HEALTHY DOGS

If you read through the above carefully, and pull out all the different foods containing all those different nutrients, you end up with a surprisingly short list of nutritious foods suitable for feeding dogs to produce maximum health, work, reproductive capacity, longevity and optimal growth. That list reads somewhat as follows...............

Animal Products
- Raw meaty bones from chicken, lamb, beef, rabbit, pork
- Muscle meat from chicken, lamb, beef, pork
- Organ meat - liver, kidneys, heart brains
- Eggs, especially the yolk
- Cheese and cottage cheese, yoghurt, milk, butter
- Seafoods - any fatty fish, herring, salmon, sardines etc.

Plant Products
- Fresh, green, leafy vegetables such as spinach, outer leaves of lettuce, cauliflower, broccoli, brussel sprouts, etc.
- Corn, sweet potatoes [the yellow ones], pumpkin, squash etc.
- Mushrooms Root vegetables, potatoes, carrots etc.
- Fresh and dried fruits - any of them Legumes - peas and beans, baked beans etc.
- Whole grains including brown rice and oat flakes, wheat germ, wheat bran, wholemeal bread

Miscellaneous
- Brewer's yeast, kelp powder or tablets , molasses

Oils
- Cod liver oil, corn oil, soyabean oil, wheat germ oil, cottonseed oil, safflower oil, sunflower oil, peanut oil

From that very simple array of commonly available foods, you can devise a diet for dogs that will make and keep any dog healthy, active, fertile and long lived.

The next chapter deals with the importance of separating and combining these foods.

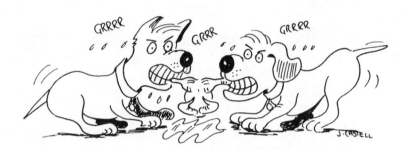

The Importance of Food Separation [and Combination]

At this point I would like to develop and discuss the idea of food separation and food combination. In human nutrition, much emphasis is placed on food combining by folk such as naturopaths. They claim that certain combinations of foods are more easily utilised by the body, and utilised without causing problems. On the other hand, certain combinations of foods "fight" each other.

This brings us to several related issues that affect the health of your dog. These include the idea of a complete and balanced diet at every meal, and the idea of mixing nutrients together and cooking them.

These two ideas are part of the "commercial dog food feeding programme". They are also part of the idea behind feeding chickens or pigs in cages, and lot feeding beef cattle. So entrenched have these ideas become, that it is now assumed by most vets, and therefore most modern dog owners,that this is the correct way to approach the formulation of meals for animals, including companion animals.

However, normal feeding of anything, including humans, does not work on the theory that every meal has to be balanced. It seeks balance over a period of time. Most meals for most creatures will consist of a limited number of food items. Never will each meal be "complete and balanced".

• Let me give you some examples of this method of eating or feeding at work in nature......

When a wild dog or a modern dog fed in a primitive way receives it's nutrition, each meal is likely to be different in size, timing, and content. It will certainly not be complete or balanced.

One meal may be totally vegetarian, e.g. the guts of some herbivore. That meal will have very little protein and no minerals whatsoever. Another meal may be all protein, e.g. some muscle meat. Another meal may be mostly liver and kidneys and other internal organs. Another meal may be mostly fat. Another meal may be mostly minerals as that dog chomps on and consumes some bones that have been stripped of meat.

Over a period of weeks to possibly months, that dog's diet is balanced. This approach to eating is in stark contrast to the way modern dogs are fed using the so called "complete and balanced diets" produced by dog food companies.

The need for each meal to be complete and balanced is the notion we get from a quarter century of feeding dogs artificially on prepared dog foods. [Longer in the United States and Great Britain]. Commercial dog foods are formulated that way through necessity, not because it is a good way to feed an animal. It is the only way they can sell their product.

However, you are not trying to sell dog food to an unsuspecting public. You are trying to feed your dog in such a way as to keep it healthy, which is a totally different thing.

Dogs, like any other animals, do not require that each meal be complete and balanced. The attempt to do that causes numerous problems. The normal, natural, and far superior way in terms of ease of doing and maximum health for your dog, is to provide the nutrients it requires over a period of time in many different meals. By doing that you will achieve superior nutritional balance and do a much better job of feeding your dog for health.

THE PROBLEMS CAUSED BY "COMPLETE AND BALANCED MEALS"

The attempt to put every nutrient an animal needs in the one cooked up product causes enormous problems for the unfortunate animal forced to eat it.

The first problem is one of nutrients no longer being available, which of course leads in turn to a myriad of health problems. This lack of availability is due to chemical interactions between nutrients when they are broken up, mixed together and then cooked.

That process results in nutrients such as calcium, chemically combining with other nutrients to produce insoluble, indigestible compounds which are no longer available to the dog. This is particularly so in commercial dog foods where excessive levels of calcium are the norm.

This situation does not occur on natural or primitive diets. Let me give a very common example. The wild dog requires minerals such as zinc, copper and iron. These will be obtained when it eats the liver of another animal. That liver will be eaten along with maybe the gut contents and perhaps with some muscle meat. It is unlikely that it will be eaten with bones which are rich in calcium. In other words, there will be no interference with the absorption of those much needed minerals.

The calcium is eaten at another meal. That is, when the dog has a bone meal. Even if bones are eaten with other foods, the digestion of the bones will be relatively slow, while organ tissue will be digested and absorbed much more quickly.

Getting back to the cooked product - the commercial dog foods - these often have trace minerals such as copper added to them. This also causes problems. The trace minerals, particularly when heat is involved, inactivate many of the vitamins.

If the food is overcooked, this produces further problems. This has the potential to produce insoluble, poorly digested compounds, for example, compounds made up of carbohydrates and proteins.

In other words, combining all these foods together and then cooking them, in an attempt to produce a "complete and balanced diet", is disasterous in terms of it's effects on the availability and usability of nutrients.

The attempt to combine all the nutritional needs of all classes of dogs from puppies to old age pensioner dogs, in the one product has it's problems as well. It eventually results in damaged kidneys because of continual excesses in the diet of protein, phosphorus, sodium and calcium.

It bothered me for a long time that the meals I advocated were often higher in protein and phosphorus than some commercial dog foods, and yet where the commercial dog foods promoted poor kidney health, the diets I was advocating did not.

The answer lies with this food separation method. Processed foods with their uniformly high protein and phosphorus levels, never give the kidneys a rest, whereas with a more primitive or natural way of feeding, where each meal is quite different, the kidneys are alternately worked and rested. One day the kidneys are dealing with a diet high in protein and phosphorus, the next day they are not.

It is the rest period, when protein and phosphorus in the diet is low which is benefitting the kidneys... preventing kidney degeneration... promoting kidney health.

Another problem is digestion and assimilation. For reasons not fully understood, greater health is obtained when foods containing mostly starch are kept separate from foods containing mostly protein.

The meals I describe further on in the book, separate predominantly starchy foods from predominantly protein foods. The original research from which these ideas stemmed was actually done with the dog.

ACHIEVING BALANCE OVER TIME

Many people find it difficult to comprehend the notion that each meal does not require to be balanced. However, we vets see this "balance over time" principle at work all the time. let me give you a very common example.

Many folk, desperate to help their dog suffering severe health problems such as infected, itching, smelling, oozing eczema, often make drastic changes to their dog's diet to see if that will help the problem.

Not uncommonly, the change will be from a processed food to an all meat diet. However, it is just as likely that the diet change will go in the opposite direction. No matter which way it goes, there will always be an improvement – for a while. You see, no matter which direction the change in diet takes, they take their dog from one poor quality diet to another, but for a while, during the period of change, the dog is closer to receiving a balanced diet than it ever has been before.

This is not because the two diets are mixed together. Commonly the change is abrupt, one day one diet, the next day the other. What they are seeing is the balance over time effect.

What these folk observe, is that for a period of several months, their dog is much healthier than it used to be. Not perfect, but much better. This convinces them that they are doing the right thing by changing their dog's diet. That the new diet is ideal.

However, after a few more months have passed, that dog will begin to develop a new set of problems, caused once again by an incorrect diet.

Of course I am not saying it is necessary to balance your dog's diet over a period of many months. For an adult dog, balance will normally be achieved over a one to three week period. For a growing puppy, balance should be achieved over say a three to seven day period.

RAW MEATY BONE BASED DIETS FOLLOW THIS PRINCIPLE

Without knowing about these ideas, many of the early feeding trials I carried out actually followed those principles, and doubtless contributed to their success.

Feeding whole foods tends to make it very simple to stick to the basic ideas behind food separation and combination, particularly because the foods are not cooked.

The most obvious food separation involves bones. For both practical reasons and for reasons of food separation, it is best to feed the raw meaty bones separately to everything else. If you try to feed a mixture of vegetables and meat, most dogs, particularly dogs that have not eaten this way before, will separate the veggies from the meat, and only eat the meat.

In the section on practical feeding, I outline a number of meals which you may use to supplement the the raw meaty bones. Each of these meals follows the ideas of separating predominantly starchy meals from predominantly protein meals. No meal attempts to be complete and balanced.

What I would like to emphasise at this point, is how difficult it is to provide balance in your dog's diet by attempting to make each meal a balanced meal. It is one of the reasons commercially fed dogs do so badly. On the other hand, it is absurdly easy to achieve a healthy balanced diet for your dog by feeding a wide variety of foods, with each meal being different. It means less thinking, less worrying, and a dietary regime which is almost impossible to unbalance. This is in stark contrast to commercial dog foods, which have their balance so easily upset.

So let me stress one more time, it is not each meal that has to be balanced as the makers of the commercial dog foods are forced to do. [not very well of course] It is the over-all eating habits of your dog which require to be balanced. This is most easily achieved by a wide variety of whole foods.... fed at different times.

[Note also that balance is never achieved by offering your dog a wide variety of brands or types of dog foods. By feeding different brands and/or types of commercial dog food, you are offering your dog what amounts to "more of the same".]

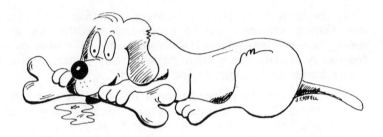

Dogs Eat Bones

This chapter contains the key to understanding how dogs should be fed. Read it carefully.

The central message is that if a dog is to become and remain healthy, it's diet must be based on raw meaty bones.

Most people know almost instinctively that dogs love bones. They have seen dogs eat them, fight over them, bury them and dig them up later on.. all rotten and smelly and decomposing.... and delicious - if you're a dog.

Despite that almost instinctive common knowledge, many modern dog owners are reluctant to feed bones. Some believe bones are dangerous. Others find them inconvenient, either because dogs fight over them, or because they ruin the garden with ceaseless burying of and searching for .... bones.

- As a result, dogs, which for tens of thousands of years have relied on bones as the most important part of their diet are suffering health problems at all stages of life, in innumerable ways.

ARE BONES DANGEROUS ?

That question is uppermost in many people's minds. The answer is ... yes, but only if they are cooked.

- DOGS ARE NOT DESIGNED TO DEAL WITH COOKED BONES.

Cooked bones are harder, more brittle and more splintery than raw bones. They are the ones most likely to be caught in the mouth, to pierce the intestines, to set like concrete in the large bowel, or to stick like fish hooks into the rectum. All those events are bad news for dogs.

The long and the short of it is... Don't feed cooked bones. They are unnatural and a danger to dogs.

Raw Bones are Completely Different !

Whilst cooked bones are potentially fatal for dogs, raw bones, in my experience, and in the experience of numerous dog owners, dog breeders and other veterinary surgeons, have been the only single food item that guarantees a dog will have excellent health. This is hardly surprising. It's a dog's heritage.

- The vast majority of healthy dogs that I have known professionally and otherwise, were bone eaters. No matter what else they ate, the central theme of their diet was raw meaty bones. By contrast, most of the sick dogs I have known, rarely if ever ate bones.

I have also noticed that there are fewer health problems in country dogs, compared to city dogs. I attribute this in great measure to the sensible attitudes towards feeding dogs exhibited by many country people, in particular the fact that they view it as normal to feed their dogs bones.

ALL MODERN DOGS ARE CAPABLE OF EATING BONES

Dogs are scavengers. For millions of years, dogs have cleaned up the remains of other animal's bodies. Mostly bones. That ability remains. All modern dogs easily and joyfully tackle bones.

- A dog's whole system is designed for and in fact needs bones to function properly. That desire and ability has not been removed from any breed of dog, no matter how altered it's mouth and teeth may be, and no matter how frail and "non-dog-like" it may look.

This includes the shortest-faced Pug dog, the daintiest Papillon, the sweetest Pomeranian, through to the roughest and toughest of Pit Bull Terriers. Any breed you care to name can, will and should eat bones.

- Age makes no difference. So long as your old dog still has sufficient healthy teeth left, eating bones with all it's benefits should either continue, or commence as part of it's life.

Your vet may have to scale some teeth, remove others that are rotten and perhaps treat your dog with antibiotics to fix a mouth infection, but once that poor sore mouth has settled down, your dog can commence to chew bones.

DOGS KNOW THAT DOGS EAT BONES

Ask any puppy whether dogs eat bones. The answer comes back in a flash.... most certainly... and don't you try and take it off me!

Ask any adult dog. We do, constantly. The answer is always the same. Yes thankyou and can I have some more please ?

Time and again, dog owners assure me that their dog will definitely not eat bones. Not long after they have come to stay with us, their dogs, even if they have never eaten bones before, are happily crunching away on their bones, and feeling so much better.

YOUR LOCAL FRIENDLY BUTCHER KNOWS THAT DOGS EAT BONES.

Talk to a few butchers. Every day they peddle bones to people for their dogs.

Recently, butchers have been advertising a product called "trim lamb". This lamb has no bones or fat. The advertising in the magazines finishes up with an unhappy dog gazing sadly at the lamb with no bone...and the words... "no bones... a disaster!"

If only dog owners could know how true those words are !

WHY ARE BONES HEALTHY FOR DOGS ?

The question you must be asking yourself is .. why are bones good for dogs ? What is it that bones have which cannot just as easily be supplied in another way ? This is a most important question.

When I began feeding my dogs this way about nine years ago, I was amazed at how well they did. I found that most dogs could eat practically one hundred percent raw meaty bones, and remain in perfect health.

This included growing puppies. They survived and grew normally. In fact much better than puppies fed the modern way on processed food and calcium supplements. In other words, as incredible as it sounds, raw meaty bones appeared to be a complete food for a dog. If not totally complete, then pretty close. I was pleased. It suited my lazy nature. It also left me a little perplexed. Why was it so ?

I have spent the last eight years or so researching that question - amongst others.

What follows are some of the answers I have found regarding bones. Why bones play such a unique and irreplaceable role in providing the bulk of a dog's nutrition, and at the same time, making dogs both happy and healthy.

I have no doubt that there are lots more reasons than I have managed to discover. However, I have found enough to convince me of the supreme importance of bones as the bulk of a dog's diet. I hope you feel the same way.

Bones.. Essential Nutrition For a Dog

Most people think of bones as something for a dog to chew on. Something which will keep a bored dog occupied for a few hours. A pacifier. The more advanced folk know that bones clean teeth. However, what most dog owners don't realise is that bones are also full of vital nutrients for their dog.

Bones are living tissue composed of living cells. Because bones are living tissue, just like any other part of the body, they are a complex source of a wide variety of nutrients.

Bones contain minerals which are embedded in protein. They also contain fat. With the fat are fat soluble vitamins and the central part of most bones contains marrow which is a highly nutritious mix of blood forming elements, including iron. Raw bones also provide natural anti-oxidant/anti-ageing factors including enzymes.

Bones Provide Your Dog with all the Minerals it Requires

Bones are nature's storehouse of minerals for your dog. They contain calcium and phosphorus in perfect balance, together with all other minerals essential for your dog's normal functioning. Isn't that beautifully simple ? No need for any mineral supplements.. just feed raw meaty bones !

- The ability of bones to provide a dog with it's complete supply of minerals is unique and irreplaceable.

For example, it is the only logical way to supply a puppy's complete and balanced supply of calcium, phosphorus and other minerals. No more guesswork. After all, that is how nature has done it for the last million years or so.

This is well demonstrated by modern attempts to raise puppies on processed foods and calcium supplements. The results of these attempts walk through vets' doors daily.

- Some are older dogs with arthritis. Lots of people think they have raised their dogs well on artificial calcium, but they are wrong. Their dog shows no obvious signs when it is young, but in later life develops one of the many forms of arthritis.

- Others are young dogs with growth problems, particularly defects in bone growth, the most popular one being hip dysplasia, but there are a host of others including OCD [osteonchondritis dissecans], wobbler syndrome, dropped hocks, splayed feet, bone cysts and so on.

If those names are unfamiliar to you, don't worry. They are not important. What is important is that puppy owners realise that every one of those modern skeletal diseases of dogs is a direct result of poor nutrition. Commercial dog foods plus calcium supplements. They do not occur when a dog is raised properly on raw meaty bones.

We have been breeding Great Danes and Rottweilers on and off for years. The bone problems our dogs had been experiencing disappeared the moment we began to raise our puppies on a bone based diet.

- That is why I stress daily in my practice that when feeding puppies, do not use calcium supplements. No matter what the breed. In fact, the larger the breed, the more important it becomes NOT to add calcium supplements to the diet, but to make sure those pups are raised on heaps and heaps of bones. As a rule of thumb, about sixty percent of the diet should be raw meaty bones.

People who heed this advice raise pups bounding with health, including perfect bone formation.

Protein in Bones

The protein extracted from bone by steam under pressure is gelatin, a poor quality protein, deficient in a number of essential amino acids.

Fresh bone is different. It contains all the essential amino acids in adequate amounts with the exception of methionine. The amino acid lysine, essential for normal bone growth is present in large quantities.

Fortunately methionine, the missing amino acid is found in abundance in meat. This means that raw meaty bones contain your dog's total protein requirements. Keep that in mind next time you feed meaty bones to your dog !

Essential Fatty Acids in Bones

Essential fatty acids are essential for perfect health. Raw bones contain fat. If the bone is from chicken [or pork], then that fat will be very high in the essential fatty acids.

Beef and lamb bones have fat which is low in essential fatty acids. By feeding lamb bones you will usually supply more fat and therefore more essential fatty acids than beef bones.

Fat Soluble Vitamins in Bones

The fat soluble vitamins A, D and E are stored in bone with the fat. This is another reason why dogs that eat plenty of raw bones are so healthy. Remember, the fat soluble vitamins are associated with enhancing the immune system and promoting healthy longevity.

- Note that when bone is cooked, these vitamins leave with the fat.

The Marrow in Bone

When your dog eats bones, your dog is receiving many of the nutrients which help produce blood and a healthy, well functioning immune system. This is because the bone marrow is where blood is formed and it is also part of the immune system of an animal. When your dog eats raw bone, he or she is consuming all the important blood forming nutrients, particularly copper and iron. Cook the bone, and many of those valuable nutrients are lost.

Energy in Bone

Because bone is full of fat and protein, it is full of energy for your dog. Note, in very fat dogs, bones are still a necessary part of their diet and should be fed daily. However, this should be in limited amounts, because of their high energy content which will help promote obesity.

The Nutrients in Bone ..... Summary

In summary, when your dog eats a raw bone, your dog is receiving high quality protein [only one essential amino acid missing], the very best mineral supplement possible, essential fatty acids if the bone is from chicken or pork, the fat soluble vitamins A, D and E, the blood forming elements in the bone marrow,including iron and copper, energy [in the fat and protein], together with the unknown factors present in all raw food.... health enhancing factors, including anti-oxidants and enzymes.

- What I am describing here, is very nearly all the nutrients your dog requires ! The only nutrients missing are some of the B vitamins, and the amino acid methionine. All you have done to get this magnificent nutrition into your dog, is to feed your dog a raw bone !

If you add meat to this diet, that is, feed a raw MEATY bone, you supply methionine and most of the B vitamins. Note also that dogs manufacture all the B complex vitamins in their large bowel, and also vitamin K.

By now you should be starting to understand why dogs can be fed raw meaty bones as the major part of their diet. Why pups can be raised on a bone based diet. Why older dogs with sound teeth stay healthy on a bone based diet. Why pregnant and lactating female dogs do their work so easily on a bone based diet. Why male dogs have no problems with infertility on a bone based diet. Why working dogs run all day on a bone based diet. Why most dogs can live almost entirely on this food for most of their lives and be healthy.

Nutritional Value of Different Bones

All bones are pretty much equal with regard to protein and mineral value. However, beef and lamb bones are very low in essential fatty acids, while chicken and pork bones are excellent in this respect.

Nutritional Value of Cooked Bones

Do remember that as soon as they are cooked, apart from becoming dangerous, bones lose much of their nutritional value. This includes the essential fatty acids, any fat soluble vitamins, many of the anti-oxidant/anti-ageing factors including enzymes that may be present, and much of the protein. The minerals in the bone are changed in a way that makes them far less useful than when the bone was raw.

Buried Bones

We all know that dogs bury bones, saving them for later on. In the case of raw bones, they slowly decompose under the action of their own enzymes. It is quite healthy for your dog to eat these buried bones... so long as it was a buried RAW BONE. It is nutritious for your dog. It just has different qualities to fresh bone. We are not sure at this stage of all of them, but they are similar to aged meat.

With cooked bones in which all the enzymes have been destroyed, the resulting rotten bone could possibly make your dog sick. Buried cooked bones cannot decompose under the action of their own enzymes. Their enzymes have been destroyed by the cooking process. Instead, they are attacked by bacteria, which can produce dangerous toxins. Perhaps the worst of these would be the toxin released by the bacteria which cause Botulism, a deadly paralysis

- Incidentally, if your dog is burying it's bones, that signals a lack of hunger..... you are over doing the feeding bit !

Bones and Dental Health

It is not hard to pick the dogs that eat bones. They look and act healthy. The acid test however, is to look in their mouth and smell their breath.

I do this daily as part of a routine examination of all dogs that enter my practice.....

Another clean set of teeth ! No sign of tartar, nice healthy gums, and doggy breath that does NOT smell like a sewer. I can say with complete confidence to this client.... "I see your dog gets plenty of bones !" ..... I have not been proven wrong yet.

Bones are Nature's Toothbrush for Dogs

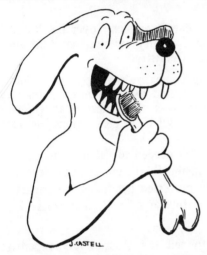

As dogs chew on bones, rip the flesh off bones, crush bones, that very action cleans the teeth, and massages the gums, stopping tartar, gum infections, tooth root decay, dental abscesses, and a whole body poisoned by a grossly infected mouth. An extremely common condition in today's dog fed on soft mushy convenience food.

Bone eating should commence when puppies are first introduced to solid food. We use minced up chicken wings and chicken necks... bones and all. After about ten days, those pups are eating the wings in their entirety, without the need to be broken up at all. Now those wings are acting as toothbrushes.

Thirty years ago, Aussie dogs did not have the dental problems they have today. The rise in the incidence of mouth problems has parallelled the increase in consumption of processed food, together with the decline in consumption of raw meaty bones.

The result of no bones on a dog's menu, processed food only, is teeth covered in TARTAR, receding gums, tooth root decay, and the most vile, stinking mouth infection.

Left untreated that mouth infection, spreads via the bloodstream, and may lodge in other organs such as the heart, lungs, kidneys, prostate, uterus etc..

Meanwhile think of the poor suffering animal, a lifetime of cruel pain..... plus rejection by an owner who cannot stand the smell.

Doggy Dentists ..... Only New in Australia

The rapid increase in canine dental problems over the last ten years has spawned a growing specialty within the Australian Veterinary profession. Veterinary Dentistry.

In 1991/92, a veterinary drug company, with expensive dental machines to sell to Aussie vets invited two American Veterinary Dentists to Australia. The idea was that these Yankee vets should persuade the Aussie vets what a great money-making racket is Veterinary Dentistry.

- Apparently, we Aussie vets needed to catch up to our American counterparts. In the States where dogs never see a bone and eat only processed pet foods, Veterinary Dentistry provides vets with one third of their gross income.

The company's aim was to sell the Aussie vets expensive dental machines. Machines that are so sophisticated, they would make a human dentist proud. More importantly, that equipment would make it's new owner a fortune ! Those filthy infected mouths, the direct result of processed foods, were literally filled with gold. All an astute veterinarian had to do was be willing to invest a few thousand dollars in dental equipment and learn how to use it !

As part of their sales pitch, those American vets tried to tell or sell us on the idea that dogs should not be fed bones... ever.

Such provocative statements raised the ire of a number of practical Aussie vets, who knew the importance of bones to the dental health of dogs.

- Since that time there has been much debate amongst vets, about the importance or otherwise, of bones to a dog's dental and general health.

The question has been asked "do dogs chew their food ?" This has lead to further questions such as... "is it bones alone, bones plus scraps of meat, or is it bones plus their full complement of flesh which clean dog's teeth and massage their gums ?"

From such learned pontificating has come the suggestion that this is an area worthy of research. That may well be so. But from my point of view it seems like an incredible waste of money to research something so painfully obvious.

My observations tell me that all of those activities are healthy for dogs. Any researchers who enter this field will be staggered at the difference they see in the health of bone eating dogs compared to the "mush-and-dry" brigade.

In the meantime, while we wait for this scientific research to prove beyond all shadow of a doubt what we already know, let us not deny our dogs the benefits of bones.

Fortunately, much valuable ground has been made within the profession out of these discussions. More and more vets have become aware of the importance of bones to a dog's dental and general health.

Many are realising that should the Australian dog-owning public start feeding their dogs bones, this new specialty [vet dentistry] within the Australian Veterinary Profession, might quietly fade away, leaving redundant a lot of expensive equipment and training.

Disappearing Dentistry

Prior to recommending bones as an essential part of a dog's diet, I had had to deal with masses of revolting, stinking, disease-ridden mouths, just like every other vet. Gradually, as my clients took my advice and fed their dogs bones, that unpleasant job was on the wane. The result was that as Veterinary Dentistry began to flourish in Australia, I was scaling down my vet dentistry activities.

These days, the bulk of my dental work is carried out on the pets of new clients. This usually involves, getting rid of the tartar from the teeth, removing the badly diseased teeth, and clearing up the mouth infections with penicillin and flagyl or whatever antibiotic is appropriate.

After that, I talk to the owner about diet, dentistry, teeth and health. Within a couple of weeks most of these dogs are confirmed bone eaters with no more dental problems and a vast improvement in health.

Meaty Bones Provide Incredible Exercise For Your Dog

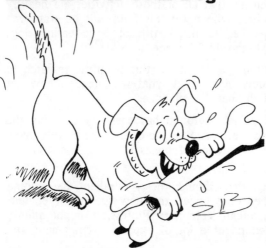

Do not cut your dogs meat up, and do not cut it off the bone. Feed it in large lumps left on the bone. This gives your dog something to do with its jaws and teeth and whole body.... exercise.

Meat left on the bone means your dog will have to rip, tear and chew at it. This is the way nature intended your dog to eat. It is part of keeping your dog healthy. It is vitally important for your dog's health that it eats it's food in as natural a form as possible. All that exercise of chewing, ripping and tearing at large lumps of bones and meat is of benefit to dogs of all ages.

It helps a growing dog to develop properly, and it helps keep an adult dog fit.

Think of a dog with both feet planted firmly on a lump of meat still attached to it's bone. Head down, taking hold of that meat, ripping and tearing away. What is that dog exercising ?

That dog is exercising it's whole body. It's jaws, it's neck, it's shoulders, and it's front legs. It is also exercising the back and hind legs which are braced to resist all this activity up front.

That process is of vital importance to growing dogs. Young dogs deprived of bones, NEVER have the correct development of their jaws, neck, shoulders, front legs, chest, back, hips, in fact their whole body ! Time and again I see weak spindly looking pups coming in to be vaccinated. They are about twelve weeks old. They have legs like chooks. Long, thin and no muscle tone. I know immediately that this pup does not eat raw meaty bones as a major part of it's diet. I know that this pup is being raised on some horrible sort of canned mush or one of the dried dog foods.

Pick the Puppy Raised on Bones

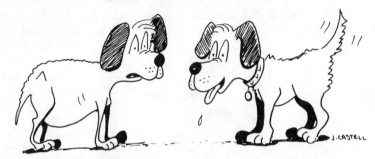

Puppies MUST Eat Bones !

It is vital to the future structural health of all dogs that they are involved daily in this form of eating exercise. The lack of healthy growth promoting eating exercise in pups, is a major part of the process which results in the bone diseases common in modern dogs.

I remember back to my early days in practice, when a client who bred the most beautiful corgis complained to me about poor shoulder development in her pups. She was concerned about poor angulation, and poor muscle tone.

I had no answer back then. Today, I have owners of corgis [and other breeds], who feed their pups as I advise, asking me if it is normal for a dog's front end to be so well developed ! When they get in the show ring, the judge certainly assures them it is OK !

Older dogs deprived of eating exercise simply grow weak and flabby. You know what they say..... use it or lose it !

Meaty Bones and Digestion

In addition to exercising and healthily stressing a dog's muscles and bones, all that ripping and tearing at big lumps of meat … on or off the bone, helps with a dog's digestion.

That preliminary activity, that hard work, sends a series of messages which alerts the entire digestive system to the fact that food is on the way. This gives the digestive system plenty of time to get ready, and do an efficient job of digesting, absorbing and retaining what is eaten.

The bone eating dog contrasts strongly to a dog fed it's food in a minced up, soft and soggy dollop. One or two gulps and it's

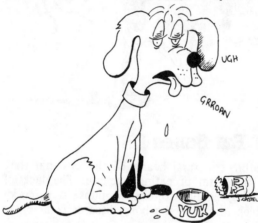

gone. No work is required. The poor creature does not even have to go to the bother of standing up to eat. There is very little time for messages to be sent to alert the digestive system which remains unprepared. This mass of mush, slides past tartar covered teeth which have not had to chew food for years, arriving as a leaden, lifeless lump in an unprepared stomach. Poor digestion, indigestion, and quite commonly diarrhoea is the result.

A few hours later, and the dog, initially uncomfortable from this amorphous mass sitting in its stomach, is now hungry once again. This is a sure recipe for obesity.

Puppies and adult dogs fed raw meaty bones rarely if ever suffer from indigestion or diarrhoea. Dogs fed raw meaty bones produce smallish quantities of solid minimally offensive stools. These are quite different to the revolting mounds of evil smelling partially liquid waste which oozes it's way out the back end of dogs fed processed food.

Meaty Bones and Your Dog's Psyche and Immune System

Ripping and tearing at it's food is very emotionally satisfying for a dog. A dog's whole being longs to eat in this way because of it's evolutionary background of hunting and scavenging. That is why eating this way is a tremendous stimulus to the immune system, and no doubt is another reason for the incredible health and disease resistance of bone chewing dogs.

Bone chewing dogs are also found to be much more evenly balanced emotionally. In contrast to what many people think, bone eating dogs are the ones least likely to be savage. It is as if they have taken out all their aggression on the meaty bones. Eating this way also means much less destructive behaviour.

Emotional balance, skeletal health and all round good health due to a healthy immune system is part of the reason modern zoos feed their carnivores on whole raw carcases rather than use processed foods. The processed foods were tested and found wanting years ago.

Meaty Bones and Obesity

A major benefit of feeding the meat in large lumps, or on the bone, is that it takes the dog longer to eat it's food. This helps with the obesity problem. It gives the dog's internals a chance to tell the dog it has had enough, BEFORE it has over-eaten.

Many people notice that after a few days on this type of food, their dog will appear to lose it's appetite. Their immediate reaction is to worry that something has gone wrong. That their dog no longer likes the new diet. That their dog is sick. Not so. In fact things are perfect. For the first time in it's life that dog is no longer hungry. It is actually satisfied.

When this happens, the very worst thing you can do is assume your dog no longer likes the new diet and go back to feeding him or her the old way on commercial dog food or whatever.

Be patient. Do not offer any food at all for twenty four

hours. Your dog WILL eat again ! If you are impatient and go back to the old food, this is a sure recipe for producing obesity and all the other disasters stemming from not eating raw meaty bones.

The other thing to keep in mind is the need for variation. For example, if you have been feeding only chicken bones for the last couple of weeks, switch, and feed some beef and/or lamb bones. The reason for the variation is not simply to please your dog. It is for the very sound reason that different meats have somewhat different nutrient contents. Variation is healthy. That is why nature builds that desire for variation into all creatures. It ensures balance in the diet.

Bones May Have a Similar Role to Fibre

It is highly probable that bones play a similar role to fibre in a dog's body. That is, a role of bulking out the food, and a role of removing toxins and promoting bowel peristalsis [movement] and general bowel health.

The possibility of toxin removal would help to explain why bone eating dogs are so healthy, and rarely [or never in my experience] suffer from cancer, while non-bone eating dogs suffer the whole range of degenerative diseases... including cancer.

Bones, Worms and Anal Sac Problems

Not feeding bones to dogs sells an awful lot of worm tablets, and good quality worm tablets are not cheap !

When our dogs ate mostly processed dog food, we often found worm eggs in their faeces. Naturally we would then worm them. From the time they ate whole raw foods, including heaps of bones, they were rarely if ever "wormy". I concluded from this that processed dog foods do not feed the immune system properly the way fresh whole foods do.

Another reason that non-bone eaters get wormed regularly is because they spend a lot of time scooting their rear ends along the ground or the carpet in an attempt to empty their anal sacs. This makes their owner think they have worms.

Sometimes their dog will have a tapeworm infestation which will cause this. More commonly, their dog's bottom is not so much itchy as uncomfortable. Their dog has full anal sacs.

What are anal sacs ? They are two little stink sacs embedded in the ring of muscle which keeps your dog's anus closed. They are full of rotten, smelly, thickish, semi-liquid to liquid material. It smells something like very off fish. Both of these anal sacs open to the outside through a tiny duct. These little stink sacs are designed to expel their contents either when a hard lump of faeces passes through the anus on it's way to the outside, or when your dog is frightened.

They are scent-cum-identification- cum- warning glands for dogs. When you see a dog sniffing another's faeces, he or she is looking for this particular signature.

If a dog has a fright, the whole contents are expelled, and all the other dogs get the message that something awful has happened or is about to happen.

If your dog does not have many frights, and if your dog does not have hard faeces, these sacs fail to empty, and become very

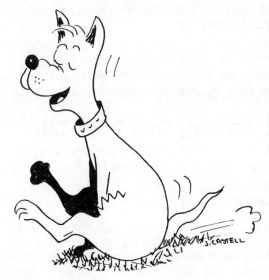

full. Your dog then scoots his bottom along the ground or the carpet, in an attempt to empty them.

If you feed your dogs lots of bones, those beautifully hard feces that result, cause the anal sacs to empty.... your dog does not have to scoot... you don't think your dog has worms... and so you save money ... not buying unnecessary worm tablets.

Note also, that anal sacs which are not emptied regularly by the passage of hard faeces, often become diseased and have to be removed. A most unpleasant operation for your dog.

All of this can be avoided by feeding raw bones daily to your dog.

Bone Feeding, Constipation and Dog Logs in the Back Yard

To a person who has fed a dog on processed food all it's life, the passage of faeces formed from bones can make a dog look as though it is constipated. When a dog has to strain to pass a nice solid faecal lump formed from bones, that is completely normal. Stop worrying !

By the way, who gets to pick them up at your place ? The "dog logs" in the back yard I mean. Not a pleasant job is it. If your dog eats lots of bones, the job will be at least less unpleasant, if not more pleasant.

The "dog logs" passed by dogs eating processed food stink. They are mushy, the canned variety stain the concrete, and those from dry dog food, because they are so indigestible, produce stinking voluminous wet faeces.

Feed your dogs copious quantities of bones and hey presto... The droppings are far less smelly, there are less of them, they are easy to pick up, they do not stain the path, and they are less likely to squash between your toes.. should you be barefoot.

Raw Bones Prolong Your Dog's Life

• Bone eating dogs are long lived healthy dogs. They seem to be particularly free of the degenerative diseases of old age.

I can see a number of reasons for this.

Firstly, the bones themselves produce all those wonderful benefits we have talked about, including dental health, good nutrition without excesses or deficiencies, proper digestion, proper development of puppies and great exercise throughout life. In addition, being raw, the bones provide all the wonderful benefits of raw food, including enzymes, and age fighting anti-oxidants.

Not only that, people who are prepared to feed lots of bones to their dogs, seem to have plenty of good old fashioned common sense when it comes to feeding dogs. They see the dog as a dog, with doggy needs, and are usually not seduced by the claims of dog food manufacturers.

They almost always feed both themselves and their dogs lots of healthy foods. That is, they feed the scraps of their healthy foods to their dog[s]. In addition, I usually find that these common sense healthy people also make sure that their dog does not become overweight !

WHAT SORT OF BONES SHOULD WE BE FEEDING OUR DOGS ?

In our hospital and at home with our own animals, we have fed every conceivable type of bone to every conceivable type of dog. All raw. In our experience with feeding bones to dogs, it is a very safe procedure. We have fed dogs this way in complete safety, over many years, as have thousands of our clients.

I must also confess, that with our own dogs that eat bones all the time, we have occasionally slipped in the odd cooked bone. However, we do not recommend the feeding of cooked bones.

From this wide circle of bone feeding experience we feel confident to offer the following comments, information and guidance.

"Dinosaur" Bones

These are the great big bones. The big long bones out of both the front and hind legs of cattle.

They are all fairly hard tough bones. That is one of the reasons I recommend them least of all.

In the past, many vets have said give only these big bones to your dog because he or she cannot break them up. The idea being, that if they could not be broken up, they would be safe.

However, in our experience, all bones are safe so long as they are not cooked. They are a dog's natural food, and may be fed with confidence.

Not only that, big dogs can break up these bones, They can chew them, and they swallow them. I am very pleased to report

they have never in our experience caused any problems. Of
course for little dogs that cannot break them up, the disadvantage is that they do not get to eat the bone, except perhaps the
softer ends, thus missing out on the nutritional aspects of the
bone. In other words, for all except the bigger dogs, these big
bones act more as pacifiers and teeth cleaners, and less as sup-
pliers of nutrients.

Many folk get their butcher to cut these big bones in half
lengthways, so as to allow the dog access to the marrow.

The main problem they do cause, because they are so big,
thick and hard, is the wearing down and the breaking of teeth.
Loss of teeth is serious, and can happen if they are the only
type of bone offered.

Actually, I do have another objection, but it is an objection
common to all bones. The horrible crunching noise that goes on
all night under the bedroom window, making human sleep well
nigh impossible.

Meaty/Boney Off-Cuts From the Butcher.

Most butchers, and this includes butchers in the major supermarkets will supply bags full of boney off-cuts. These off-cuts
will vary as to the proportions of meat bone and fat, and of
course as to the beast they came from [either lamb or beef
usually], and finally as to which bones are included. That is,
they can contain all sorts of bones - eg. chop bones, beef ribs,
necks, backbones, the pelvis - etc.

We do do not try and sort them out, mostly accepting whatever bones are there, and dolling them out to all and sundry. At
our place, all and sundry includes Rotties, a fox, a Bull Terrier,
some cats and Toy Poodles, plus a number of client's dogs that
are staying with us as we correct their nutritional problems.

The only sorting we might do is if we feel there is too much
fat on a piece for our fat little poodle. We do sort out the mea-
tier pieces for the cats, and the softer bones for any young pups
we are raising.

• We think of these off-cuts, as good general bones. They

keep dogs happy, their teeth clean, and as described,
supply much of their nutrition.

We have NEVER had any problem from these bones with our
dogs, or dogs that have had bones from birth. In fact we have
RARELY seen problems with raw bones – period.

I have seen rib bones, raw ones, caught in the mouth between the teeth. However, I do not see that as sufficient reason
for recommending against bones. They are not difficult to
remove, and their presence is always obvious... for eg. drooling,
difficulty eating, general discomfort etc. etc.

These bones are obviously wedged tight – use a pair of pliers
or multigrips to remove them. The only thing you may possibly
need to be alert for would be infection in the mouth if the bone
pierced the gums or palate etc. If that were the case, your dog
may need a shot of penicillin or some other antibiotic as your
vet decides.

Chicken Bones

Raw chicken, on the bone is without doubt the very best
form in which to feed your dog most of it's requirements of raw
meaty bones.

Most people, when I suggest they feed their dog chicken
bones [I often recommend chicken wings], reel back in horror and
surprise... and say.... "But I thought you were not supposed to
give chicken bones to dogs ..... ! ???"

The answer is of course, that it is most certainly not a good
idea to feed COOKED chicken bones to your dog.

I can remember my first case of cooked chicken bones. I had
been in practice only a short time. My son David had a little toy
Poodle. Her name was Elizabeth. That poor little soul had got in
to the garbage can. She had polished off a whole heap of
cooked chicken bones.

Those darned things were hard and sharp, and they were
stuck in her rectum, each sharp point jagging into her rectal
wall. She was in agony. Fortunately, not hard to fix, but I never
forgot the danger of cooked chicken bones.

There is an incredible difference between cooked and raw chicken. Have you ever tried to chew on raw chicken ? It is TOUGH. The bones on the other hand, coming from ten week old birds are extremely soft. Once your dog has crunched through that flesh, the bones are very safely crushed. Contrast this with cooked chicken. The flesh is beautifully soft, while the bones have gone brittle and sometimes quite splintery. These are dangerous ! DON'T FEED COOKED CHICKEN BONES TO YOUR DOG.

- Since discovering the joys of feeding chicken to dogs, raw chooks have become the most popular item of food on our dogs' menu. They have in fact become the mainstay of their diet.

We pop along to a chook processing plant where they bone out the chooks to make all that lovely human chook fare such as chicken kiev and boneless chicken stuffed with apricots etc. etc.. What we pick up are the chicken carcases, the boned out chicken legs, necks and various other bits and pieces of chook at an incredibly cheap price.

This is the waste which is normally processed to become commercial dog food, or chicken mince. In its raw pristine state, straight from the factory, not processed, not cooked or minced, with no chemicals or preservatives or coloured dyes added, it is incredibly valuable food for our dogs.

Chicken pieces, the carcases, the wings, the necks, whatever, I now consider to be the most important raw meaty bone for our dogs. There are a number of reasons for this.

An obvious and important reason is their availability. Because chicken is now a major human food, and much of it is being deboned, it is freely available at bargain basement prices. Some chicken outlets are even paying people to dump it !

Of all the meaty bones available, chicken carcases would undoubtedly be the most nutritious and the safest. The chickens from which they come are exceptionally young... two to three months at the most. The bones are soft and have no toxins. Chickens do not carry hydatid tapeworms.

DOGS OF ANY AGE CAN EAT THEM !

- Raw meaty chicken bones can be fed to the very old, the very young, the very sick, in fact to any dog at any stage of life.

They have the best essential fatty acid content of all animal bones. They are beautifully balanced with respect to their bone to flesh ratio, and when raw, they are soft and safe. This is why wings and necks are so good for puppies. Plenty of bone for their bones. The wings are a rich source of bone marrow, rich in blood forming iron.

- Chicken protein is of exceptional quality with respect to essential amino acid content and is easily digested.
- Chicken bones are a brilliant way to introduce bones to the old, the young and the never-had-bones before animal.
- Chicken pieces, especially chicken wings make an excellent basic diet for lactating mums. They have all that protein and calcium so necessary for producing lots of rich milk for the pups.

They provide all the other valuable assets of bones as I have already outlined.

Raw Chicken Carries Bacteria

Raw chicken does of course carry bacteria, E.g. - Salmonella. Also Campylobacter jejuni. These are of absolutely no consequence to a healthy dog. However, after handling raw chicken, [and remember you do this all the time when you prepare a chicken meal for the family], wash your hands before eating, and sterilise all utensils, implements and cutlery etc. used in it's preparation. It's that simple.

FEEDING OLD DOGS, YOUNG DOGS AND TOOTHLESS DOGS ON BONES

And also dogs that have never eaten bones before. We introduce bones into the diets of all these animals by mincing up chicken wings or chicken carcases or whatever bits of boney chicken bits we have.

If initially the dog does not like the taste, we mix a tiny portion of this minced chicken with a larger portion of whatever it does like... also minced. Over a period of time, we gradually increase the proportion of minced up chicken bits. For more information on how to encourage your fussy dog to try new food sensations, refer to Chapter 20.

BONES YOU SHOULD NOT FEED

Do Not Feed Your Dog Cooked Bones

Many dog owners have real horror stories to tell about feeding bones to dogs. Things such as anal piercing by little spicules of cooked chicken or chop bones. Bones that have pierced their dog's bowels, bones that have become caught in the mouth, throat, oesophagus etc. At the time, it caused their dog a lot of grief and cost them a lot of money. That is why I am never surprised that they vow never to feed their dog, any dog, a bone ever again.

- However, what must be borne firmly in mind is that almost every problem caused to dogs by eating bones has been caused by COOKED BONES.

Rule number one is... do not feed cooked bones to your dog. Feeding cooked bones is a little like playing Russian roulette. You may get away with it for years, or you may have a disaster straight away.

I have met folks who have given their dog cooked bones for it's entire life with no problems. Others, myself included, feed cooked bones to their dogs - occasionally... again no problems. However, if any bone is going to cause a problem it will be the cooked bone. From the moment people began feeding their dogs cooked bones, there have been problems. These multiplied at a rapid rate once the idea of cooking food for dogs became firmly entrenched in people's minds.

Why are Cooked Bones so Bad ?

The obvious answer is that they are a totally unnatural way to feed a dog. For the last million years or so dogs have been eating raw bones. That is what their body, their digestive system is geared to handle.

I have already mentioned the physical changes in bones that occur following cooking, however, they are very important and deserve repeating. Cooked bones are harder, more brittle and more splintery. They are the ones most likely to be caught in the mouth, to pierce a bowel, to set like concrete in the large bowel, or to stick like fish hooks into the rectum.

Bones, once cooked are very poor nutritionally compared to raw bones. Their whole chemical composition has changed. They become very much like any other processed unnatural food. Their protein is of MUCH lower quality. Not much different to gelatine. They have lost most of their fat, and therefore their essential fatty acids and their fat soluble vitamins. The marrow, once cooked is much less valuable nutritionally.

Having lost their rawness, bones have lost their enzymes, all the vitamins which are destoyed by heat, and all the anti-oxidants and other anti-ageing factors in raw foods.

One of the most important changes that occurs is to the minerals in that bone. It is probable that the calcium in the bone chemically combines with other minerals in the bone making them unavailable. Cooking the bone changes the way your dog's body assimilates the calcium in bone. It behaves like any other ARTIFICIAL source of calcium, resulting in problems relating to an excessive intake of calcium, causing problems in both growing and adult dogs.

- The bottom line on COOKED BONES is DO NOT FEED THEM TO YOUR DOG.

Avoid Feeding Bones from Older Animals to Your Dog

Bones from older animals have a number of draw backs. They are much harder than bones from younger animals. This means that they will be very wearing on your dog's teeth, and may even result in a broken tooth.

Old bones store toxins. The older the animal, the more toxins that will be stored in it's bones. For example, an old cow kept pastured in a paddock near a main highway all it's life will have bones full of lead from leaded petrol fumes. Not a great idea to feed these to your dog. As I mentioned earlier, when you buy processed dog food, you take all sorts of risks including the strong possibility that such toxin-filled bones went into the mix.

These days it is not common for older animal's bones to end up in butchers shops. If they did, they would most likely be beef bones. As beef bones are also low in essential fatty acids it would be better not to feed large old beef bones to your dogs, particularly if you are able to choose an alternative.

- The bottom line is, where possible, feed bones from young animals.

Bone Meal - a Good Idea or Not ?

Within the last fifteen years in Britain, bone meal as a source of calcium for women afraid of developing osteoporosis, had to be banned. Much of this bone meal had been derived from old carthorses which had spent all their lives in city traffic, concentrating lead from petrol fumes in their bones. Some of these women languished in mental institutions until it was realised that they were suffering from lead poisoning.

What about bone meal for dogs ? I do not recommend it. Bone meal is ground up and cooked bone. In other words it really is only cooked bone, without the physical dangers but with all the nutritional problems of cooked bones including the very real possibility of some sort of toxicity, including chronic lead poisoning.

BEEF, LAMB, OR CHICKEN BONES ?

Beef ?

In sum, beef bones are probably the ones you should avoid if you have the opportunity to do so. They MAY be older, they will probably be harder, they may have more toxins, their fat is low in essential fatty acids, and they usually have the least amount of flesh left on them.

Lamb ?

Lamb bones are probably the most common ones that people are able to get hold of. They can be very fatty, and that is something to be avoided in some instances. Cut the fat off, or simply throw away the really fatty pieces. Lots of dogs do very well eating lamb flaps. Occasionally we find an animal that cannot tolerate lamb. It seems to cause diarrhoea. In that case, switch to chicken.

Lamb bones as the name suggests come from a young animal. The bones are soft with few toxins. The essential fatty acid content is reaonable because of the high fat content, and there is usually a reasonable amount of meat left on them.

- The one drawback with any raw lamb products is the possibility of hydatids [see Chapter 9]. However, this is certainly not a problem if you purchase them from a butcher.

Chicken ?

In terms of nutritional quality, safety, their contribution to dental, and therefore general health, freedom from hydatids, easy availability and their cheapness, these would have to be the best type of bone to feed to your dog.

Some larger dogs will get into the habit of swallowing chicken carcases whole, which means that many of the benefits of bone eating are denied that dog. For that reason, and because variability is important when it comes to feeding dogs, it is wise to also feed both lamb and beef bones on a regular basis.

Many people myself included feed rabbit, pork and even fish bones.... all raw, and with a good covering of raw flesh of course, to their dogs and have absolutely no problems. We just get very healthy dogs.

Incidentally, rabbit is quite a good food for dogs if you can get hold of it. It is a valuable food for dogs with bad skin due to eating dry dog food. It has a good balance of essential fatty acids.

HOW MANY BONES SHOULD I FEED MY DOG - AND HOW OFTEN ?

Bones should be fed DAILY to your dog, That's right.. every day. At the very least, feed them three times a week. Any less than that, and all the problems kept away by bones gradually start to appear. For example, tartar starts to build up. Tartar build up usually means that junk food is creeping in. Once the rot sets in, dog owners become lazy, they forget to go to the butcher, and gradually bones are fed less than once a week, then hardly at all. In other words.. keep the habit up. Keep feeding your dog bones, or you will lose the habit, and your dog will suffer.

Please also note that I have been emphasising the words raw and meaty. Please do not just feed bones without the meat. At the same time, do not feed meat without bones. What I mean by that is do not feed all bones without meat all the time, and do not feed all meat without bones all the time.

Remember, it is what you do for most of the time that counts. In other words, a meal of pure bones now and again is fine, just as a meal of pure meat is fine now and again. Just do not let one or the other idea take over and become the way it is always done.

- Remember also that an all meat diet is a disaster. Don't do it. Similarly, an all bone diet, that is, bone without meat even if it is a raw bone diet, can result in a bowel blockage [severe constipation] and DEATH.

FEED BONES WHEN ?

Lots of people are not sure when to feed bones. Often, if feeding bones AFTER other food, the dog says..."No thanks, I am too full, I am saving these for later on... so I will now proceed to bury them..."

For that reason it is probably best NOT to feed bones when your dog is full from other food. We feed bones to our dogs when they are hungry.... mostly, but we also feed them if they have had a small amount of other food, just to leave them with something to do .. keep them occupied for the rest of the day.

BALANCING UP A BONE MEAL

Actually, that is what the rest of the book is all about. The important point to grasp from this chapter is the unique and fundamental importance of raw meaty bones to dogs. The fact that raw meaty bones should form the bulk of the diet, somewhere between forty and eighty percent, depending upon what else you decide to feed.... and on that point I advise you to keep reading.

- 8 -

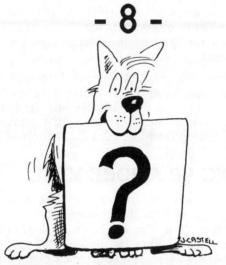

Feeding Meat to Your Dog

FEED THE DOG MEAT - A GOOD IDEA OR NOT ?

In this chapter I explore the role of meat as part of a balanced diet for dogs. There is not really a lot to know. In short, meat supplies high quality protein. The best way to feed it to a dog is raw, on the bone, as already described. However, people ask me lots of questions about meat, so I shall start talking about it by answering a few of those questions.

Is Meat Good Food for Dogs ?

Yes, because dogs are carnivores, it is totally natural for them to eat meat, it is an excellent source of high class protein. However, even though it is excellent as part of their diet, let me stress that if meat forms the whole of a dog's diet, or most of it, that dog will eventually become sick. This brings me to the next question.....

Can My Dog Survive on Meat Alone ?

When I tell people that commercial dog food is sub-standard canine fare, and is causing their dog's many health problems, they commonly ask, "does that mean we should just feed our dog meat ?"

The answer is of course no. A meat-only diet is highly unnatural and highly unbalanced. It is in fact one of the common feeding errors I have already spoken about in Chapter 4. You will recall that raw meat is deficient in a number of essential nutrients including calcium, iodine, and vitamin C, and by itself would give a dog too much phosphorus and protein.

- An all or largely meat diet fed to an adult dog over a lifetime, with it's excessive protein and phosphorus will eventually cause chronic kidney disease, together with numerous other problems resulting from it's many nutrient deficiencies.

- For a growing puppy, the calcium and iodine deficiencies cause immediate bone and growth problems. These surface in as little as two weeks. An all meat diet was the most popular way to wreck puppies, particularly their bones, about fifteen years ago in Australia, but is less common these days.

Other frequent questions are as follows.

Should Meat be Cut up or Left in Large Lumps ?

Meat off the bone should definitely be left in large lumps. It is far better for dogs to have to rip and tear and chew the meat.

Some people become concerned when a dog regurgitates a large lump of meat. However, resist the temptation to remove it from your dog. Watch while your dog either chews it a little more thoroughly, or swallows it whole again more carefully, more slowly.

Is it Essential for Dogs to Eat Meat ?

Definitely not. Your dog might be a carnivore, but he or she being an omnivore, can quite happily exist without meat. In fact, if your dog does eat meat, it should only form a small part of the over-all diet. Dogs have not evolved to eat muscle meat as the major part of their diet. The muscle meat eaten by wild dogs forms a small part of a diet that consists of a wide variety of other foods, including a lot of bone.

Should My Dog's Meat be Cooked or Raw ?

For your dog's sake, the meat should be raw. Raw meat has all the benefits of raw foods as discussed in chapter two.

Dogs have always eaten it that way. Raw meat is one of the foods your dog's body is designed to use. Cooked meat is not. Raw meat has innumerable health promoting advantages. Cooked meat given long term promotes failing health.

- Over-cooking meat decreases protein digestability and destroys essential amino acids such as lysine and methionine. A common example is poorly processed pet food, particularly dry dog foods. Here it is common for over-cooking to make a poor quality product even worse.

Cooking can appear to have advantages. It can help to remove fat, but is it worth it when you can use a knife ? Also, the mineral levels in meat cooked on the bone are higher than in raw meat because they leach out into the meat from the bone. However, a dog is far better to eat the meat AND the bone - raw. That way your dog has access to ALL the minerals.

- IMPORTANT - read Chapter 9 which deals with the disease HYDATIDOSIS which can be transmitted from dogs to man via raw meat.

A lot of people tell me they will not feed raw meat to their dog because it will encourage their dog to take baits. Unfortunately, many a poisoned dog has been killed by poison placed in cooked meat and other cooked food.

What Nutrients are in Meat ?

Meat Supplies Protein.

That is it's major role in nutrition. It also supplies varying amounts of fat, water, and some vitamins and minerals. Because it supplies fat and protein, it also supplies energy.

- MEAT PROTEIN IS FIRST CLASS PROTEIN.

That is, it contains all the ESSENTIAL AMINO ACIDS necessary for dogs of all ages, including growing dogs, pregnant dogs, female dogs feeding puppies, and of course desexed-living-at-home-not-doing-very-much-dogs.

The protein is of high quality because it is very DIGEST-IBLE in contrast to the protein from vegetable sources which is much less available for your dog.

Chicken and pork, the white meats are somewhat lower in protein content than sheep and beef. Beef has the highest out of these four.

Meat Supplies Fat

The fat in different types of meat varies in the level of essential fatty acids present. Chicken and pork have the highest levels while lamb and beef are both low. Lamb usually contains more essential fatty acids than beef, but only because it has more fat.

Meat Supplies Water

Lean young meat is 70% - 75% water, with the rest being mostly protein. Meat from older animals contains less water. Note that canned dog food contains on average, more than 80% water.

Meat Supplies Energy

There are no carbohydrates in meat. That is, no starch or sugar or fibre. As the fat content rises, the percentage of water drops and so does the protein. As the fat content of the meat rises so does the energy it can supply your dog. For example, a lean piece of meat weighing 100 gm will contain about 400 to 450 kj of energy. If that same weight of meat consisted of 30 percent fat, it would supply three times as much energy.

That extra energy is great if your dog is working hard. If not, it will cause obesity.

Meat Supplies Minerals

- Raw meat is low in sodium and high in potassium.

This is good news for older dogs with heart problems. The meat with the lowest sodium is beef, with pork also being fairly low. The meat with the highest potassium is pork, with chicken having the lowest potassium levels.

This makes lean pork a good all round meat for heart patients, particularly in view of the high levels of the amino acid Taurine present in pork. Taurine is essential for normal heart function.

- Beef, sheep, chicken and pork meat are all very low in calcium and moderately low in magnesium.

This means they are great foods for dogs prone to bladder stones. However, let me stress that this lack of minerals in meat requires that your dog eats bones as well as meat.

- Both beef and sheep meat are relatively well endowed with zinc, making them good foods for dogs with a deficiency of zinc.
- Unfortunately chicken has low zinc levels. Pork has more zinc than chicken but not as much as sheep and beef.

- Of the meats, beef is probably the best source of iron, with sheep next, then pork, with chicken coming last. If your dog is consuming whole raw chicken wings it is getting iron from the bone marrow.

Meat is NOT a Complete Food

It is valuable to know what meat does not supply. Meat is deficient in some of the B vitamins, vitamin C, calcium, iodine, copper, vitamin A, vitamin E and vitamin D.

Pork contains no vitamin A at all. Chicken fat has more vitamin A than any of the others, with beef coming second and sheep having very little. The general lack of vitamin A in meat is easily remedied with either a vitamin A supplement such as cod liver oil, or some liver once a week.

Pork has the best levels of vitamins B1, 2, and 3, with chicken having the lowest.

So far as cholesterol is concerned, chicken has the highest levels, with beef having the lowest. Pork and sheep are intermediate for cholesterol.

- Unless you have a reason to know the above details, forget about them. The reason I include them is to help you realise the importance of feeding a wide variety of meats to your dog. That is, feed some of each ... not all at once, at different times will be fine. By doing that you will ensure a better balance of all those various nutrients present at different levels in different types of meat.

Is minced Meat any Good for My Dog ?

Minced meat is not natural, so that in most instances it is less valuable than meat fed whole - on the bone.

Firstly, all the physical benefits are lost. That is, meat that has been minced means no ripping, tearing, chewing, teeth cleaning, gum massage etc.

The other problem is, unless you minced the meat yourself, you really have no idea what is in it. You do not know what ingredients were used, and you do not know what chemicals have been added. You have lost control over your dog's food.

Unless you minced it yourself You also have no idea of the original state of the meat, and whether it was prepared hygienically. Particularly mince sold as pet food.

Having said that, let me add that problems caused by contamination are not common because of a dog's natural ability to eat bacteria-laden food. When problems occur, it is usually the very young and the very old or the already sick. That is, animals whose immunity is not working one hundred percent effectively.

Minced meat is of value however when changing diets. The new minced-up diet is thoroughly mixed with the old minced-up diet. It is also valuable for young puppies as a small part of the diet, or for old or sick dogs, or dogs with no teeth, as part of their diet. Get it from a reliable butcher or mince it yourself.

- Note that raw mince is better value for your dog than cooked mince.

How Much Meat Can or Should My Dog be Fed ?

The amount required depends very much on the age and activity of the dog.

For an adult dog who has finished growing, so long as he/she is eating bones as at least 50% of the diet, then from nothing up to half the rest of the diet could consist of meat with the rest being fruit and/or vegetables and/or cereals and/or organ meat etc., plus vitamin supplements. For more information on practical diets for adult dogs, puppies and older dogs, please turn to the appropriate chapter.

Which is the Best Sort of Meat to Feed My Dog ?

The choice in Australia is between, beef, sheep, pork and chicken. In pet shops you will also be able to purchase meat labelled as horse, kangaroo and buffalo. However, in many parts of Australia, MOST of the red meat you buy in pet shops is kangaroo, even if it is labelled otherwise.

Although meat generally contains first class, good quality protein, the one exception is horse meat where the quality and digestibility of the protein is lower than other meats. There is not much difference between the more commonly used meats in this respect. However, out of beef, chicken, lamb and pork, beef is highest and chicken is lowest.

The major difference between meats is in the level of ESSENTIAL FATTY ACIDS. Chicken and pork have the highest levels, with lamb second, beef third and kangaroo last. I have no data on the horse, except that most of it is pretty lean, but the fat which is present is yellow and oily, indicating the presence of carotenoids [vitamin A precursors] and high levels of unsaturated fats.

Kangaroo meat is very lean. The protein is of excellent quality. I have no reliable data on the type of fatty acids present, although I would suspect they fall somewhere between beef and sheep on the saturated side and pork and chicken on the unsaturated side.

As your dog ages, the white meats are far more healthy for dogs than the red meats. From a scientific standpoint I am not at all sure why that is so. I do not know whether it relates to the level of essential fatty acids present, the lower protein, or some unknown factor. It is just that the red meats seem to be associated with more degenerative conditions such as arthritis.

Rabbit as Dog Food

Whole rabbits are great food for dogs. They are a very natural food for dogs, and of course are a complete food, containing everything your dog needs, including good levels of the essential fatty acids.

- We feed them to our dogs whole, both with the fur removed or left on. Our dogs particularly love the heads which are rich in nutrients because of the brain and the eyes.

In greyhound circles it used to be common to feed a whole

rabbit to a not-one-hundred-percent-well greyhound, particularly a greyhound with diarrhoea which could not be attributed to any specific cause.

Raw Beef Meat as Dog Food.

Beef is very popular as dog meat. It is an excellent source of high quality readily-digested protein. Beef contains higher levels of protein than sheep chicken or pork. It usually has less fat and therefore less energy than the other meats which means it contributes less to obesity. It has the lowest cholesterol levels but is low in essential fatty acids, with 5 % polyunsaturated, 47 % monounsaturated and 48 % saturated fat.

Beef is very low in calcium. It has good levels of iron and zinc. Chuck and skirt steak have the highest zinc levels. This is important when male dogs have reproductive problems or when dogs of any description have skin problems.

Beef contains small amounts of the B vitamins [1, 2 and 3], but very little of any of the others.

- When dogs are fed mostly beef, they seem to have more health problems than when lamb or chicken is fed. I am not sure why this is so.

It may be due to a lack of minerals because beef is usually fed without bones. Both chicken and lamb are usually fed on the bone, or if fed cooked, even without the bone, the meat and juices contain the minerals which have leached out of the bone during the cooking process.

It may also be due to a lack of essential fatty acids.

Another possibility is that beef off the bone does not clean the teeth and provides no eating exercise. Most dog owners make matters worse by cutting the beef up into small pieces.

- Greyhounds often perform best on beef.

This may relate to it's high protein, zinc and iron content, and the fact that any deficiencies in vitamins and essential fatty acids are made good with incredibly high levels of supplementation. It may also relate to the fact that some of the more successful grey hound breeders/trainers feed beef in the way that wild dogs eat beef. As the whole animal.

Greyhounds fed this way have to work for their food. They have to rip and tear it off the bone. They eat the innards including organ meat, the grassy contents of the bowels, and the contents of the large bowel, which is rich in essential fatty acids and B vitamins. They also eat it as it "goes off"... which confers other nutritional advantages to a dog whose whole evolutionary history is filled with eating in this manner.

Contrast that to most other dogs fed beef today. Almost invariably, it is without the bone attached. Certainly the rest of the carcase is not available as a source of nutrition.

Raw Sheep Meat as Dog Food

Lamb is very "fatty". Fat can make up to thirty or forty percent of what you feed, even more with fatty off cuts from the butcher. The cholesterol levels are slightly higher than beef.

The excessive fat can be a problem. If that is so, either cut it off, or don't feed that excessively fatty piece.

The fat is only 3 % polyunsaturated, with 54 % saturated and 43 % monounsaturated.

- Because lamb is often fed untrimmed, it supplies more essential fatty acids than beef.
- Zinc in sheep meat varies from 2 to 10 % but is mostly about 3 to 5 %. This is similar to beef. The highest levels are found in the shank and the neck chops. If your dog has a zinc deficiency, these are the cuts to feed.
- Because lamb supplies plenty of fat as well as zinc, switching dogs with skin problems from a dry dog food diet to a diet based on lamb, meaty off-cuts often sees a dramatic improvement. More so than switching to beef with it's lower fat levels.

Note that a lamb shank has only 2 % fat, so do not rely on lamb shanks to fix fatty acid deficiencies.

The protein levels in lamb vary betweeen 15 and 32 %, depending mainly on how much fat is present. As fat increases, the protein levels drop. This protein level is slightly lower than beef.

Like any other raw unprocessed meat, sodium is low and potassium is high. That means sheep meat may be fed to dogs with heart and kidney problems. Note that lamb shanks are higher in sodium than other cuts.

Calcium levels are a bit higher in lamb than in beef, but still too low to feed a lot of lamb without bone. Do feed the bone! Iron levels are quite reasonable, just slightly less than beef but better than chicken.

The levels of vitamins in lamb are roughly comparable to beef.

- The bottom line with sheep meat, particularly if it is on the bone, is that it is valuable dog food. This includes shanks, breasts, chops, legs, shoulders, ribs, necks, pelvis, backbone, head etc..

We have fed all of these pieces over many years to many different dogs with few problems. Occasionally we notice, and clients report, that some dogs suffer diarrhoea when fed sheep meat. The simple answer is not to feed such dogs with sheep meat, or introduce it slowly to minimise digestive upsets.

Raw Chicken Meat as Dog Food

- We find chicken is the best all round meat for our dogs.

Naturally we always feed it on the bone – as nature intended. It makes up about sixty percent of the raw meaty bones we feed our dogs.

- It can be the fattiest meat fed to dogs, particularly when feeding boned out chicken carcasses as we commonly do.

Fat can be anywhere from 3 % to 40 %. Of the fat, 14 % is polyunsaturated, 52 % is monounsaturated and 34 % is saturated. In other words, raw meaty chicken bones are an important source of essential fatty acids, and also of the protective monounsaturated fat. Chicken has higher cholesterol levels than beef.

- Protein is lower than in beef lamb or pork. It ranges between 13 and 28 %, but most cuts contain between 20 and 25 % protein.

Chicken has lowish sodium, with about three times as much potassium. Like other meat, it is low in calcium and magnesium.

- Compared to beef lamb and even pork, chicken flesh is low in iron and zinc, particularly when it is fed raw.

Like all other meats, as soon as you cook the meat on the bone, some of the calcium and iron and zinc leach out into the flesh.

- Compared to the other meats, chicken is much higher in vitamin A, but still does not have enough to satisfy all your dog's requirements. It has adequate levels of the B vitamins, with no vitamin C.

We feed raw chicken on the bone to all sizes and shapes and ages of dogs. Raw chicken wings form the basis of our small dogs' [Poodles and Miniature Foxy's] diet. Most owners of toy breeds will testify to the great gusto with which small animals attack chicken meat. Unfortunately, most of these people feed COOKED chicken and no bones.

- Our big dogs often get whole chickens !

Two lady clients were very lucky. I did not have to go into any great explanation. I was telling them about the importance of chicken wings, and while they were going through the usual shock-horror-gasp reaction, without saying a word I ushered them into the room where we keep our canine boarders.

On that day we had a female Miniature Foxy with five four week old puppies staying with us. They had just been fed. Naturally they had received chicken wings. Mother was eating with great gusto, crackle and crunch as she chewed through those bones. The little ones were tackling theirs with no less enthusiasm, just a little more difficulty. They were making sufficient headway for those two ladies to be totally convinced that this unheard of concept was entirely possible.

They like many hundreds of other dog owners went home and tried the chicken wings on their own animals, with the usual outstanding success. They experienced trouble free acceptance of the wings by their pets, and the rewards that followed in terms of the greatly increased health of their little dogs.

Warning !

Please note... COOKED chicken bones should not be fed to dogs because they are dangerous ! Cooked, and therefore hardened and brittle chicken bone cased in soft cooked chicken flesh is a potential danger to any dog. It can cause problems anywhere along the dog's digestive tract, and it often does. Feed RAW chicken, on the bone !

For young, small and old animals, or animals whose teeth have seen better days, I recommend using a cleaver or meat mallet to break the bones into small manageable pieces. Do this in such a fashion that the skin is left mostly intact. I often rub brewer's yeast into this.

If you must feed cooked chicken to your dog, remove the bone.

Hormones in Chicken ?

A lot of people believe that chicken meat is full of hormones and will therefore cause problems. This worries breeders in particular. I have not found this to be a problem. The use of female hormones in Australian chickens was outlawed years ago because of the potential dangers to human health.

There is no reliable data confirming or otherwise the possibility that chicken meat may contain some form of growth promotant with hormone like activities. What I can tell you however is that in my experience, with both my own animals, and talking to numerous breeders who have switched their dogs to a raw chicken-meat-plus-bone based diet, there have been no problems. On the contrary, we have all been delighted with healthy, happy dogs that are reproducing beautifully.

Pork as Dog Food

Not a lot of people feed pork to their dogs, except perhaps the folk who go out pigging. If that is. you, please read thoroughly the section on hydatids. Pork is excellent meat for dogs having a good balance of essential fatty acids, good quality protein which is high in the essential amino acid Taurine, and very high in the vitamins B1, 2 and 3. All other vitamins are largely absent.

Total protein will vary from 15 to 30 %, with protein mostly running at about 20 to 25 %. That is, more than chicken but less than beef or lamb.

Total fat varies a lot, as it does in chicken, from as low as 2 % on a very lean piece of meat, up to 30 % or more. The fat is made up of about 12 % polyunsaturated, fatty acids, 51 % monounsaturated and 37 % saturated. That is, it is quite like chicken. It has good levels of the essential fatty acids.

The cholesterol in a lean piece of pork is more than beef but less than chicken. As soon as it is grilled or baked, the cholesterol rises.

As with other meats, there are no carbohydrates in pork. There is a good ratio of sodium to potassium with about five or six times more potassium than sodium.

- Calcium is low as it is in all meat.

The level of zinc is better than in chicken but not as good as lamb or beef. Pork contains virtually no vitamin A.

Pet shops and Pet Meat

If meat is purchased from a pet shop, there is the risk of buying meat to which identifying dyes and chemical preservatives have been added.

Pet shops rarely or never, sell meat on the bone, the preferred way to feed meat to a dog.

- The sort of meat offered for sale can vary, but over the years I have seen labels proclaiming the meat to be any one of beef, buffalo, chicken, horse, and kangaroo. Despite these labels, much of the red meat sold in pet shops is kangaroo.

Kangaroo Meat

Kangaroo is very lean and sometimes requires added fat. For example mutton, or better still chicken fat or pork fat - lard. I recommend the chicken and lard because of the higher levels of essential fatty acids.

Buffalo Meat

I can only assume that buffalo meat is much the same as beef, quite nutritious, but low in essential fatty acids, so that both buffalo and beef based diets require added fat or oils rich in essential fatty acids.

Horse Meat

Most horse meat is very lean, which makes it lower in energy than other meats. It is also less digestible than other meats. This will often lead to diarrhoea. If feeding horse meat, do not feed a lot of it, feed some other meat as well, e.g. chicken or mutton or fatty beef.

Chicken Meat From Pet Shops

- This is usually sold minced. Unfortunately, all the comments I made above about other forms of minced meat apply. That is, the dog loses the exercise and teeth cleaning effect of eating whole chicken, and you lose control over what is in the food.

If the source is reputable, fresh chicken mince containing bones is a valuable food. It is a good way to introduce a dog to raw chicken ... whole. However, of all the processed pet foods available, this is the one most likely to contain harmful [to your dog] bacteria. We never buy it, preferring to feed our dogs on chicken carcasses.

If you do buy chicken ready minced from a pet food supplier, check to see whether it has had preservatives added, and if so what sort. If they are of the anti-oxidant type, particularly if it is vitamin E, that is far better than none at all. Anti-oxidant preservatives stop fats going rancid - a basic cause of many long term health problems in dogs. Unfortunately, some dogs are allergic to preservatives and will develop eczema diarrhoea and other problems when when forced to eat them.

- The bottom line is that anything sold in a minced state, should always be viewed with suspicion, until proven otherwise. Mincing can be used to hide a multitude of sins.

Feeding Meat During Hot Periods

During hot weather limit the amount of meat you feed to your dog. In fact restrict total food intake. Your dog does not need it, particularly if it is overweight. If your dog is overweight, this is a perfect time to help him or her lose weight. To do this, lengthen the periods between meal times, and feed less bulk at each meal. Feed only raw fruit and vegetables. If your dog is not interested in these, then he/she is not really hungry, and will probably lose weight ! Do not coax an overweight dog to eat at anytime !

However, some dogs lose too much weight in hot weather due to excessive panting and a reduced appetite. In that case it can be important to feed more energy-dense food. That could mean fatty meat - preferably on the bone.

Handling Raw Dog's Meat

The dog's digestive system is built to handle a whole range of microbes that are of potential danger to man. We see the dog's ability in this regard every time it digs up and consumes the rotting remains of meat on a buried raw bone.

- So when handling raw meat, particularly raw chicken meat, observe sensible precautions, thoroughly washing all plates and implements in near boiling water, together with the usual personal hygiene things like thoroughly washing hands before consuming your own food.

Feeding Fish to Your Dog

Fish can form a small part of a balanced diet for your dog. If you feed a lot of it, you must make sure you feed the whole fish with it's entrails, eyes etc., and do make sure you are giving plenty of vitamin E supplement.

However, my broad recommendation is do not feed a lot of fish to your dog. As part of a mixed diet it is fine. One type of fish I would recommend on a regular basis would be sardines .. mixed in with some other food. The benefit here is you are supplying your dog with some of the omega 3 group of essential fatty acids.

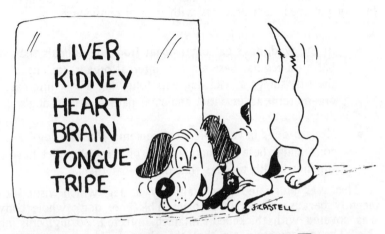

Organ Meats as Dog Food

USELESS OFFAL OR VALUABLE FOOD ?

Because it is readily available and cheap, large numbers of Australian dog owners regularly feed their dogs liver, kidney, brains, tongues, ox cheeks etc.. Butchers often put together packs of this material specially for dogs.

The question is, is this a good idea ? Are such things valuable food for dogs ? What nutrients do dogs get when they eat organ meats ? If dogs are supposed to eat this sort of food, how much should they get and how often should they get it ? What are the dangers of feeding too much organ meat to a dog ? Are there different stages of life when extra will be required ? Which is more nutritious for a dog, cooked or raw organ meat ? Is there any danger to a dog's health if it eats organ meat raw ? What about human health ?

These are the sorts of questions that people ought to be asking when it comes to feeding offal to dogs. The answers are important. By understanding what these products contain, and how they can help or possibly harm a dog, allows dog owners to feed or not feed such products with greater confidence.

- In the wild, dogs eat organ meat from the animals they kill on a regular basis. In fact internal organs are one of the first things a wild dog eats following a kill. Internal organs form an essential and vital part of a wild dog's diet.
- Modern dogs have similar requirements. Modern dogs consuming these products as part of a sensible diet have superior health to dogs that do not eat them.

This was illustrated graphically by a dog which visited us recently because of a skin problem. This poor dog's whole body was covered with thickened, inflamed, infected, oozing, crusting skin. The owners told me that the skin would often clear up, and stay healthy for months, then suddenly, the problem would reappear.

The basic diet of this dog was dry dog food. Recently it had been eating one specifically formulated to improve the coats of show dogs. Clearly the product was not doing what it's makers claimed it would !

After questioning, it became apparent that the dog's general health, including it's skin, improved whenever it was fed a product called "dog's delight". This was a concoction put together by the local butcher and consisted of a mixture of livers, hearts, kidneys, brains, tongues and off-cuts of various meats including pork and lamb and beef.

- This mixture was rich in high quality protein, B vitamins, vitamin A, some vitamin C, essential fatty acids and zinc. That particular mixture, if fed often enough, adequately compensated for the deficiencies of the dry dog food.

This is a common situation. Many folk manage to balance their dog's diet quite nicely in all sorts of ways, including the use of organ meats, without really understanding what they are doing. On the other hand, some people feed organ meat as the major part of their dog's diet. Such dog's eventually become ill.

- Obviously organ meats are valuable dog foods. But not in huge amounts. Wild dogs do not eat huge amounts. They are a concentrated source of many essential nutrients. Ideally, your dog should eat small amounts of them all it's life.

- Organ meats are particularly valuable during times of growth reproduction and stress, as a source of essential concentrated nutrients.

- The vitamins they contain include members of the B complex, vitamin A and vitamin C. The minerals they contain include iron, manganese, selenium and zinc.

- Most organ meats have excellent levels of high quality protein and essential fatty acids. They contain a lot of phosphorus, but they are very low in calcium.

As with most other foods, they are more valuable nutritionally when fed to your dog raw, containing health promoting enzymes and naturally occuring anti-oxidants, including cholesterol which also has anti-oxidant properties. It is quite probable they contain nutritional factors, anti-oxidants etc.... not yet discovered.

Do feed them on a regular basis, but do not to feed too much of them. Organ meats should only form about ten or fifteen percent of the food eaten by an adult non-reproducing, not-doing-very-much type dog. Dogs that are growing or reproducing will require more.

THE NUTRITIONAL VALUE OF DIFFERENT ORGAN MEATS

Liver as Dog Food

Liver is the most popular organ meat fed to dogs. This is hardly surprising. In this one product is a vast range of important nutrients.

Heading the list is vitamin A. Liver is the most concentrated source of this vitamin known. For example, approximately 100 gm of lamb's fry contains around 30, 000 international units of vitamin A. For it's vitamin A content alone, all dogs should be fed liver on a regular basis. It also contains vitamins E, D and K in substantial quantities.

Liver is an excellent source of the minerals zinc, manganese, selenium and iron. Most dogs fed on dry dog food, or a cereal-based canned product can be deficient in all of these. Anaemic dogs may be fed liver as an excellent source of iron. Dogs with skin problems and male stud dogs may be fed liver for it's zinc content. All dogs require liver for it's selenium content. Selenium is part of a major body anti-oxidant called glutathione peroxidase.

Liver is an excellent source of all the B vitamins, particularly B2, B3, B5, B6, biotin, folacin, B12, choline [or lecithin] and inositol. It contains B1 or thiamin in adequate but smaller amounts compared to the other B vitamins. Liver is a good source of vitamin C.

Liver is a source of good quality protein, and the essential fatty acids, both the omega 3 and the omega 6 type.

- The bottom line on liver is that by feeding it on a regular basis, you are supplying your dog with an excellent balance of a wide range of nutrients which are essential for health, including healthy skin, healthy reproduction, and healthy temperament. It is a fantastic food for your dog !

Scientists are still not sure if they have discovered all the growth promoting and health conferring factors present in this food.

- This means that it is still a good idea to feed liver even when you are supplying many of the nutrients we know it contains from other sources. That way, your dog will not miss out on important but undiscovered nutrients.

Liver contains cholesterol. A little bit less than is found in eggs. This is not usually a problem for dogs, unless the dog is extremely obese or has a particular problem with cholesterol.

Kidneys as Dog Food

Another fantastic food for your dog. Not unlike liver, they supply good quality protein, a good supply of essential fatty acids and many vitamins, including all the fat soluble vitamins, A, D, E, and K.

Kidneys are a rich source of iron and all the B vitamins including B12. They also have good levels of zinc. Their vitamin A content is good, but much less than liver. Kidneys are an excellent source of essential fatty acids.

Their cholesterol level is slightly less than is found in eggs.

Brains as Dog Food

Brains supply protein, fat and water. They have a cholesterol content of about three times as much as is found in eggs. This means that dogs with a cholesterol problem should not be fed brains. They are a good source of most of the B vitamins except folacin and biotin. Brains have good levels of vitamin C, with virtually no vitamin A and a small amount of vitamin E.

- They are an excellent source of essential fatty acids.

Brains are good brain food and good skin food.

Hearts as Dog Food

Like liver and kidneys, hearts as dog food are an excellent source of protein, B vitamins and iron. They do contain some essential fatty acids, and a little vitamin A. Their cholesterol levels are about half as much as eggs.

Tongues as Dog Food

Tongues may be thought of as a source of protein fat and water. They also supply some of the B vitamins. They are probably of not much greater value than muscle meat. They do contain reasonable levels of zinc.

Tripe as Dog Food

Not to be highly recommended. Tripe consists of protein and water with a few B vitamins. Green tripe, straight from the killed beast is of greater nutritional value to the dog because of the presence of large numbers of micro-organisms.

YOU HAVE TO BE CAREFUL WHERE YOU GET YOUR ORGAN MEAT !

Apart from the nutritional aspect of too much or too little, organ meats can cause problems of another type. The internal organs of animals like cattle and sheep can carry dangerous parasites. Parasites that will not harm your dog, but can damage human health.

* The principal danger is from the Hydatid tapeworm.

That is why, it is important that I give you the important facts on the Hydatid tapeworm and the disease it can cause in human beings.....

Hydatidosis.

* The most important point you will get from the following information is that provided you buy organ meat from a butcher, or use organ meat derived from poultry, there will be no problems. Please read on to see why.

The offal of many animals that dogs are likely to eat has the potential to contain cysts of the pathogenic [to man] Hydatid tapeworm. It is this human health aspect of feeding dogs that has been the major reason for dogs being fed cooked meat and meat products.

* The dog is the animal which transfers the disease Hydatidosis from sheep and other animals to humans.

This problem is not insurmountable however, and with a little care and understanding, Hydatidosis will be avoided. The problem is not usually seen in the city or suburbs.

- It is a disease almost exclusively of country folk, who feed sheep offal to their dogs, usually while killing sheep for home consumption.
- In recent years it has also become a problem for weekend warriors and their families and friends and neighbours. That is, the folk who take their dogs into the bush to hunt pigs and kangaroos etc..

Hydatid Disease in You and Me

The whole problem is due to a tiny tapeworm called Echinococcus granulosus. This tapeworm is only three to nine millimetres long. It's name is not important, but the disease it causes, the disease your dog can PASS ON TO YOU AND ME ... HYDATID DISEASE most certainly is.

This disease is found throughout the world. In Australia it is commonly found in farmers and their families in sheep raising areas. It has until recently been VERY UNCOMMON in the suburbs.

- The worst areas in Australia for Hydatid disease are Southern N.S.W., the Canberra area, and Western Victoria.

In Australia over all, Hydatid disease in humans occurs at the rate of about three cases per one hundred thousand people per year. In some sheep raising areas, the occurrence is ten times as much.

- Human Hydatid disease consists of cysts which form most commonly in such organs as the liver and the lungs.

It can however form in the kidneys or the heart or the spleen, in fact ANY organ in the human body. They have also been found in the head and in the bones. I do not have any figures for the Australian situation, but in England, about three people die from this disease each year. I would expect a similar situation exists here.

Why talk about hydatid disease in humans in a book which is about feeding dogs ? The answer is simple.

- Dogs that eat RAW OFFAL from sheep particularly, but also from cattle, pigs, camels, horses, kangaroos, and buffaloes, in fact from practically ANY herbivore or omnivore, can pass HYDATID disease on to human beings. There are two important exceptions. Poultry and rabbits,

Rabbits and poultry DO NOT carry hydatid disease. However, whilst offal such as the liver, from healthy birds may be fed to dogs without posing a threat to human health, rabbits can be a problem.

Rabbit Offal as Dog Food

Lots of people over the years have opened up rabbits and found a liver full of tapeworm cysts. THESE ARE NOT HYDA-TID CYSTS. They do however pose a threat to human health if your dog eats them.

This parasite is called Taenia serialis. Once again, the name is not important. What is important is that it will form cysts in humans. Your dog can pass this parasite to you. This problem is not common but it does happen. These cysts form in nervous and other tissue. The bottom line with rabbits is ..... do not feed rabbits containing tapeworm cysts to your dogs. If your dog hunts and eats rabbits, then do worm your dog as I have described towards the end of this chapter.

- There is one common misconception we should clear up. Your dog CANNOT pick up Hydatids by eating the manure from any of these animals.

Hydatid Disease ... the Details

Take yourself out to the country side. Picture a mob of sheep being rounded up by that great Aussie dog.... the Kelpie. There is a lull in proceedings, while the dog stops for a moment to go to the toilet. To defaecate. Five seconds and it is done. Back to work.

That innocent looking dog dropping just happens to contain millions upon millions of eggs from the Hydatid tapeworm. This dog has not been wormed for at least two months.

Over the next few weeks, that dog dropping will dry out. It will be trampled into the dust by sheep. It will become part of the soil and the dust, as will those millions of eggs. Some of the dust containing these eggs will end up on the grass and be eaten by sheep, or by kangaroos or by cattle or horses. Some will end up on the sheep's wool, or on THE COAT OF THE SHEEP DOG. These eggs are VERY resistant and can hang around for months. It is the eggs on the coat of the sheep dog which pose the greatest threat to human health. They are the ones a human being is most likely to pick up.

Hydatids in Sheep, Cattle, Kangaroos and Pigs etc

The eggs that are eaten with the grass by sheep or cattle or pigs or kangaroos etc. hatch out in that animal's small intestine and the Hydatid embryos enter the veins which go to the liver. Here, most of them stop.

In older sheep or bigger species such as cattle, because the blood vessels in the liver and the capillaries in the rest of the body are larger, the Hydatid embryos can continue on past the liver to the lungs and sometimes out into the general circulation where they may lodge in organs such as the kidneys, the heart, the spleen, the lymph nodes in the chest, and more rarely the pancreas, the bones and the muscular tissue.

- Wherever those embryo Hydatids decide to stay, whether it be liver or lungs or kidneys etc., they form a cyst. A Hydatid cyst. Most commonly the cysts are found in the liver and the lungs.

The shape of that cyst is controlled by the organ in which it is found. If there is no pressure on it, it is usually spherical. In the liver, which is where they are most commonly found, they will often be an irregular shape as they grow around and past the bile ducts.

After about six months, these cysts will have grown to about one and a half to two centimetres in size. They are very visible if you happen to open that animal up, and look at the infected organ.

Hydatid Cysts are very Visible !

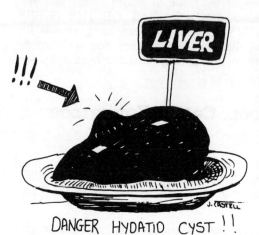

DANGER HYDATID CYST !!

In other words, if they are there, you cannot miss seeing them. If the cyst is on the surface of the liver, as they commonly are, they will be very prominent whitish cysts. If the cyst is in the body of the liver, under the surface, they will cause a prominent bulge in the normally smooth outline of the organ.

Infective Cysts

In sheep and cattle and pigs, at some stage between nine months and two years, those Hydatid cysts start to contain HUNDREDS, THOUSANDS .... MILLIONS ... of new tapeworm heads. Now they are dangerous.

- Now they are infective. In the case of wallabies, and possibly kangaroos, those Hydatid cysts may be infective as early as eight months of age.

If that animal, that cow or that sheep or that kangaroo or that pig dies or is killed, and it's liver OR ANY ORGAN with an infective Hydatid cyst is eaten by a dog, the dog becomes infested with all those new tapeworms.

- It takes six to seven weeks in a dog for those baby tapeworm heads to develop into mature adult tapeworms. This happens in that dog's intestine.
- After that six to seven weeks development, the dog is passing tapeworm eggs in it's faeces to start the cycle all over again.

- Special note.. In Tasmania, it takes only five to six weeks from the time a dog is infected to the time it is passing hydatid eggs. This is because in Tasmania, there is a different strain of Hydatid tapeworm to the one on the mainland.

Hydatid Disease in Humans

Remember the dust on the dog ? The dust that contained the eggs of our little friend the Hydatid tapeworm. Remember that sheep and cattle and pigs etc. could eat grass with that dust on it and develop Hydatid cysts in various organs in their bodies ?

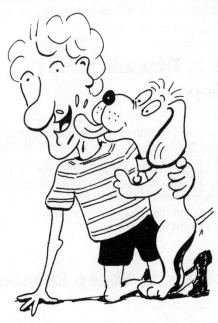

Sadly, exactly the same thing can happen with humans. Our affectionate dog, who has just licked himself, may lick you or me, or a child... on the mouth for example, transferring those eggs to us. We can pat our dog, or even one of our sheep, not wash our hands and eat something and again pick up Hydatid tapeworm eggs. In fact, patting our dog and then not washing our hands before eating is probably the most common way we become infected.

- We too will soon have Hydatid eggs hatching out in our small intestine, burrowing through our intestinal wall, and from there moving to the liver and beyond. WE NOW HAVE HYDATID DISEASE. We have caught this disease from our dog.

- Those embryos inside us do exactly what they do in sheep and other animals. They slowly grow into cysts.

The symptoms and problems caused by those cysts depend very much on the organ in which they grow, and how big they become. For example, a cyst in the eye could cause blindness. One in the brain could cause severe headaches and other symptoms similar to a cancerous tumour of the brain. It is however rare for Hydatid cysts to develop in the brain.

- The most common organs in which they are found are the liver and the lungs.
- The time it takes before symptoms are seen in humans is variable. In the case of a child, symptoms may show up within a year. In adults it often takes longer. It may take many years for symptoms to develop.

Hydatid Disease in Humans Mostly comes from Sheep

The sheep IS THE MOST IMPORTANT carrier of Hydatid disease. In sheep, about ninety percent of the Hydatid cysts are or will become infective.

Less commonly CATTLE will pass Hydatid disease to dogs. This is less common because dogs do not usually have access to beef offal and also because most Hydatid cysts in cattle are NOT infective. However, any animal that contains Hydatid cysts is potentially able to pass the disease to dogs who can then pass it to humans.

The Hydatid Problem in Sheep Raising Areas

In the bad old days, when a farmer killed a lamb for the family, or maybe an older sheep for the dogs, it was quite traditional for the dogs to hang around waiting eagerly for bits of fresh liver and other innards. Those farmers did not realise that what they were feeding their dogs might ultimately be a health hazard for humans. Usually for their families.

I would love to be able to say that practise is very rare these days. I would like to be able to say that most farmers have been educated NOT TO FEED RAW OFFAL to the dogs. Sadly, they have not. This sort of thing still goes on, both on old established farms, and also on that modern invention the hobby farm.

- Feeding Old Sheep to Dogs is Not a Great Idea.

Whilst the feeding of offal to dogs from young sheep and cattle which have not passed through a meat inspection process is a dangerous practise, even more dangerous is to let them dine on older sheep meat and offal.

The older sheep, is the one more likely to be fed to the dogs. It is also the one most likely to contain large numbers of infective Hydatid cysts in it's body. In very young sheep, the cysts may not yet be infective and it is difficult for the cysts to pass through the liver to other organs. However, in older sheep with larger blood vessels, the cysts do get through and spread to the rest of the body...including in rare cases to muscles and bones. In older sheep, most of the cysts will be infective.

- Feeding these old "killers" to the dogs... RAW... sheep that have not much other value, MAY seem a very logical thing to do. Unfortunately, it is an excellent way to spread Hydatid disease to humans.

This means that while it MAY be possible to feed RAW meat and bones and even offal from a lamb under nine months of age to your dog, and get away with it, the practice of feeding similar cuts from old sheep is a practice fraught with danger to human health.

Campaigns in New Zealand and Tasmania to eradicate Hydatid disease have been highly successful. They have involved a total ban on offal feeding of dogs, together with purging ALL DOGS to detect those dogs which are carriers. Those dogs are then of course treated.

In south eastern Australia, dogs are NOT being tested to see if they carry the Hydatid tapeworm. They ARE being wormed of course, but at the discretion of the farmer. The farmers are being educated NOT TO FEED OFFAL TO THE DOGS, and in some instances they no longer do..... OR DO THEY ?

As I have said, some farmers still feed raw offal and old sheep to their dogs. However, even if they do not do this deliberately, many farm dogs, still have access to sheep carcases containing infective Hydatid tapeworm cysts.

- The problem is dead sheep left to rot in the paddock. Dead sheep not removed as soon as they die. Combine OLD sheep carcases left to rot in the paddock with dogs allowed to roam at will and therfore having free access to such carcases, and you have a situation where the Hydatid tapeworm is still very free to infect humans.

Farm dogs eat these carcases with great delight, particularly where their regular fare is a poor quality dried dog food. They then become infected with Hydatid tapeworms, and from there they have the potential to spread the disease to any of the humans with whom they come in contact. Those dogs also continue to infect the sheep.

Leaving dead sheep lying in the paddocks also allows the dingoes, the foxes and the wild dogs to pick up the disease and spread it far and wide.

New Sources of Hydatid Disease for Humans

Until recently, it was the sheep farmers and their families who were at greatest risk from Hydatid disease. Unfortunately, a new at risk group is now recognised.

The people who go bush to hunt kangaroos and pigs together with their dogs are becoming, the next major source of Hydatid disease in the human population in Australia.

This is because their dogs have free access to dead kangaroos and wallabies when they are out in the field. KANGAROOS and WALLABIES carry Hydatid disease. This is important. Most of their cysts are fertile !

Dogs eating uncooked kangaroo offal or meat are at risk of getting Hydatid tapeworms, which means their owners and other people with whom they come in contact are at risk for contracting Hydatid disease. Pigs also carry Hydatid cysts. MOST.. but not all of the pig cysts are sterile. However, the bottom line with pigs is that like cattle, they CANNOT be ruled out as a source of this infection either.

- Of course it is not only hunters and their dogs who are at risk. ANYONE WHO LETS THEIR DOGS LOOSE IN THE BUSH IS AT RISK.

Humans Don't Have to be Involved !

There are cycles of Hydatid infection which do not involve domestic animals. This is because dingoes and foxes carry it as well as dogs, resulting in cycles between foxes or dingoes on the one hand and wallabies or kangaroos and pigs on the other.

The most likely sources of infection for foxes and dingoes are kangaroos, wallabies and pig carcases killed by dingoes or hunters. Wild dogs and dingoes are more important as a source of Hydatids because they carry many more Hydatid worms than foxes.

The Fox Problem

The fox population is becoming more numerous. This is because it is no longer being hunted for it's coat. The Animal Liberationists and other similar bodies have seen to that. As a result, it is invading the suburbs more and more in search of food, thus increasing the likelihood of spreading Hydatids to humans. This is particularly so in south eastern N.S.W.

- Where dogs are used to hunt pigs and kangaroos, the incidence of Hydatid disease in the pigs and kangaroos of that area is much increased, posing a severe threat to the local community. This disease is then being spread to adjacent sheep raising areas VIA DINGOES AND FOXES, and from there to the farming community.

The Cat and Hydatids

The cat DOES NOT carry Hydatid disease. Humans cannot get Hydatid disease from cats. However, if you feed Hydatid contaminated meat to your cat, it is always possible for a dog to steal some of it. So don't !

The Meat Inspection Service

Before meat is passed fit for human consumption at the abattoir, it must be inspected by a meat inspector. The meat inspector inspects the carcase and it's internal organs for any problems that would make it unfit for human consumption. Having passed that inspection, the meat is then able to be bought by a butcher, cut up and sold to the general public.

That means when you buy meat or offal [liver, kidneys etc.] from a butcher, you can be certain there is no danger of infection from Hydatid disease.

Freezing Meat Kills Hydatids

* FREEZING MEAT at minus 20⁰C for ten days will kill any Hydatid cysts in the meat. This means the meat is safe to feed to your dogs.

However, you must be certain that your freezer is capable of reaching such a low temperature. You must also be certain that the meat in the centre of the freezer did reach that low temperature.

Heat Destroys Hydatids

Thoroughly cooking all meat and offal makes any Hydatid cysts present harmless.

Worming Your Dog

On the mainland of Australia, kangaroo and pig hunters, or any body who feeds suspect meat to their dogs should worm their dogs with PRAZIQUANTAL [Droncit or Drontal] AT THE

RATE OF 5 MG PER KG every six weeks. In Tasmania, because of the shorter life cycle of the Hydatid tapeworm, this would have to be done every five weeks.

- If you suspect your dog has, at any time been exposed to Hydatid disease... that is, it may have eaten meat or offal that could have had Hydatid cysts .. worm your dog with PRAZIQUANTEL ... now.

THIS DOG HAS NOT
BEEN WORMED....

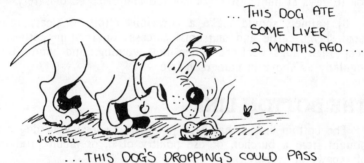

... THIS DOG ATE
SOME LIVER
2 MONTHS AGO ...

...THIS DOG'S DROPPINGS COULD PASS
HYDATIDS ON TO YOU AND ME !!

Recommendations

1] The only RAW meat or offal you should ever feed to your dog will have come from animals that have passed through the meat inspection service, [that is.. you bought this material from a butcher] or from poultry. This includes rabbits. OTHERWISE, do not feed raw offal or meat from sheep, cattle, pigs, kangaroos, wallabies to your dog[s].

2] Raw bones and meat from young sheep and cattle for your dog which you purchase from the butcher is fine for your dog. It poses no threat to human health.

3] Poultry does not carry this disease. Fresh healthy cuts of chicken [or ducks, turkeys etc.], may be fed to your dog raw with no problems.

4] With rabbits, which are excellent food for dogs, do inspect them to be sure they are free of any tapeworm cysts before feeding them to the dog.

5] If feeding your dog on food that is at all suspect with regard to Hydatids, worm your dog every six weeks [five in Tasmania] with PRAZIQUANTEL..... 5MG PER KG.

6] A SPECIAL WORD TO THE OWNERS OF KANGAROO AND PIG DOGS... and other folk with dogs that get out in the forests and bush .. these dogs are CONSTANTLY AT RISK from Hydatids.... which means that YOU AND YOUR FAMILY ARE ALSO AT RISK.... so they MUST be wormed as in paragraph five above.

7] All suspect meat should either be well cooked or frozen for 10 days at minus 20^{0}C, or not fed and disposed of safely.

8] Farmers should make a conscious effort to clean up all dead sheep, cattle and marsupial carcases on their properties, to keep their dogs confined when not working, and worm them regularly as above in paragraph five.

THE BOTTOM LINE

The bottom line is that it is quite safe to feed your dog offal bought from a butcher, or use poultry offal, or rabbit offal free of tapeworm cysts.

- 10 -

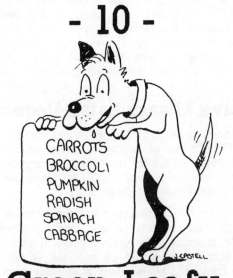

Green Leafy Vegetables - an Essential Part of a Healthy dog's Diet

Because dogs are omnivores, vegetables, particularly green leafy vegetables should form a substantial part of their diet. They are not essential however. Dogs can live and survive without such fare. There is only one problem. They will never be totally healthy. Their lives will be short, disease-ridden, and painful. In other words, vegetables are essential for a dog's health. It is impossible for a dog to be totally healthy unless it spends a lifetime eating vegetables as a major part of it's diet.

Looking at this from another perspective, while dogs cannot live successfully on a meat only diet, all dogs will thrive on a properly constructed vegetarian diet. Not that I am trying to promote canine vegetarianism. I make this point because most people think of dogs as carnivores. That is, as non-vegetable eating animals. Nothing could be further from the truth.

Dogs Have Always Eaten Vegetables

Vegetables have been an important part of a dog's diet for a long time. Country people know this. As you drive along the roads in outback Australia, it is not uncommon to see dead kangaroos, the victims of road accidents. These are quickly eaten by the local dogs, foxes and dingoes.

The first parts which disappear are the stomach and intestines together with their contents of raw, finely crushed and ground-up vegetable material. This grass/vegetation eating by members of the dog family is observed all over the world, wherever herbivbores are consumed by members of the dog family.

- The obvious questions begging to be answered are ... "Why do dogs eat this material ? Why do they need it ? What does all this vegetable material supply ? Why is it that dogs require vegetables, particularly the green leafy ones, to be completely healthy ?"

The answer is very simple. Dogs need vegetables because they contain many important health promoting nutrients. There is one nutrient in particular that only vegetables can supply. Fibre. Dogs which do not eat vegetables will miss out completely on raw vegetable fibre, which has it's own unique set of health promoting properties.

Fibre and Dogs

The fibre your dog obtains from raw vegetables includes both soluble and insoluble fibre. This fibre is quite different from the insoluble fibre derived from cooked grain, as found in commercial dog food. That insoluble fibre is much less valuable nutritionally.

The fibre found in raw vegetables is important in both preventing and treating certain diseases of the digestive tract. The so called "fibre responsive" diseases. These include obesity, most of the diseases involving the lining of the intestines, diseases involving the failure of food absorption which includes diseases of the pancreas, plus other pancreatic problems such as sugar Diabetes and Pancreatitis.

These disease problems are rife in modern dogs fed vegetable free processed diets, or home produced diets consisting mostly of grains or meat, with little or no vegetable fibre. Not only that, I predict that in the next few years, many disease problems in dogs will be found to have as their basic initiating factor, a diet low in vegetable fibres.

Vegetables Don't Only Supply Fibre

Vegetables supply many other nutrients. Many of those nutrients are the ones that have been found to be in short supply in the modern dog's "civilised" diet. This includes the difficult to obtain omega 3 essential fatty acids, most of a dog's vitamin needs, masses of enzymes and various anti-ageing factors, including anti-oxidants.

Significant quantities of the omega 3 group of essential fatty acids are present in the vegetable material eaten by herbivores such as sheep, deer, cattle etc.. In due course this material is eaten by wild dogs directly from their prey's intestines.

- As a result, wild dogs receive the omega 3 group of fatty acids in abundance. Our modern dogs do not. The result is skin problems, growth problems, reproductive problems and problems of degeneration.

Green leafy vegetables also contain most of a dog's vitamin needs. The only one they lack completely is vitamin B12. In addition, they are low in thiamin and choline. Apart from that they supply most members of the B group, that is, B2 [riboflavin], B3 [niacin], B5 [pantothenic acid], B6 [pyridoxine], Biotin and Folacin in abundance. They also supply abundant quantities of vitamin C, vitamin A, vitamin E, vitamin K and carotenoids.

- It is hardly surprising that dogs which do not eat properly
  prepared vegetables, but are maintained on cooked and
  processed foods, suffer so many vitamin deficiency
  problems. Not classical deficiency diseases, but growth,
  reproductive, degenerative and immune system diseases.

The carotenoids in vegetables are one of the anti-oxidant or
anti-ageing nutrients. In that role they are known to be
extremely beneficial in the prevention and possibly the treatment
of cancer. In addition, they are known to play a valuable role in
the female aspects of reproduction.

One of this group, Beta carotene, also known as pro-vitamin
A is converted into vitamin A in your dog's intestines, and then
absorbed. This results in a vegetable-eating dog receiving a much
greater amount of vitamin A than a dog fed cooked and processed food only. Vitamin A is essential in every process in your
dog's body.

- The vitamins A, E, C and K are all derived from green
  leafy vegetables. They are all anti-oxidant vitamins
  playing essential roles in growth, reproduction, disease
  prevention and the prevention of degeneration and ageing.

Dogs in the wild receive considerable amounts of vitamin C
in their diet because of their vegetable eating habits. This is in
stark contrast to the dog fed processed foods, which receives no
vitamin C in the diet at all. Vitamin C is the anti-stress, pro-
immune system vitamin.

- By now it should be obvious that dogs on cooked and
  processed foods are receiving food which is extremely
  poor in nutritional value by comparison to a diet rich in
  green leafy vegetables.

Processed Foods Have Very Little Useful Vegetable Matter

- The only vegetable material supplied in large amounts by processed dog food is overcooked grain.

This is a food the dog does not require. The vegetable material a dog requires in large amounts, green leafy vegetation, is completely missing.

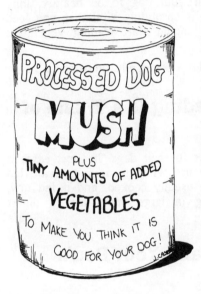

Processed foods which claim to have vegetables in them have a token amount of vegetable material only. They usually have the addition of a green dye to make the product look as though it is chock full of vegetables. Unfortunately, masses of people actually believe the dog food companies. They believe that overcooked grain, stained green with dye is doing their dogs good. Such is the power of advertising !

These comments apply equally to all the so called "natural" dog foods springing up on supermarket shelves. They too are no different to any other processed dog food, or possibly worse if their manufacturer includes the green dye.

- Naturally the poor dogs eating such rubbish are never completely healthy. They lack energy, are anaemic, and have problems with growth, reproduction, disease resistance, and ultimately degenerate into a premature, sick old age.
- The addition of green feed to such a diet would make an incredible difference. Breeders, puppy owners and the owners of elderly dogs should note this point particularly.

Vegetables Confer Long Life and Health

Modern feeding trials demonstrate that you can deprive your dog of meat and it can still be very healthy, but rarely can you get away with NOT feeding vegetables. Your dog has evolved through countless generations to require a large proportion of it's diet to be vegetable matter, particularly the green leafy type.

In other words, if you want your dog to be healthy, long lived and active into old age it is absolutely vital that you feed it raw vegetables. Ideally you should start feeding vegetables when it is a puppy.

However, unless the vegetables are properly prepared ....

Much Vegetable Feeding is a Waste of Time

Many folk do feed vegetables to their dogs. In most cases it is a waste of time. This is because when modern dogs are fed vegetables, those vegetables are usually cooked, and if fed raw, they are presented to the dog in large impossible to digest chunks.

Cooked Vegetables and Your Dog's Health.

- Your dog can digest cooked vegetables, but the process of cooking causes them to lose many of their vitamins, enzymes, anti-oxidants etc..

For example, The loss of enzymes through cooking leaves your poor dog with a double loss. Firstly, your dog's food has lost the self digesting power of it's enzymes. This puts an incredible strain on your dog's pancreas. It is a lifetime of cooked food, particularly the zinc deficient, high in soluble carbohydrates, enzymeless, commercial dog food type, that produces much of the Diabetes and other pancreas related problems.

Secondly, there are no enzymes to be assimilated into the bloodstream whole. The food has lost a major anti-ageing nutrient.

There is also the loss of the water soluble vitamins and minerals tossed out in the cooking water. Other vitamins such as vitamin B1 and vitamin C are destroyed by the heat of cooking.

Another loss is caused by the effect of excessive heat on the proteins which become denatured, or combined into useless compounds with carbohydrates.

It is also highly probable that cooking destroys many health giving properties of raw fibre.

- In other words, cooking your dog's vegetables may make it possible for your dog to get a small amount of energy, protein and a few vitamins from them, but in the cooking process, the greater bulk of the health conferring nutrients have been lost or destroyed.

Can Dogs Digest Raw Vegetables ?

Unfortunately, most folk who feed raw vegetables to their dog, feed a product which passes through undigested, making it even more useless than cooked vegetables.

This is because most of the raw vegetable material fed to modern dogs is fed in large chunks. It has not been broken up and crushed. Even grated vegetables are not of much value to dogs. In other words, if you are going to feed raw vegetables to your dog, for any value at all to be obtained from them, they must be properly prepared. That is, totally crushed !

When a herbivore such as a sheep, goat or kangaroo eats grass or any other vegetable material, they chew it into tiny pieces and they crush it. It is only when the vegetation has been "processed" [dare I use the word].... in this way, that it is suitable fare for a wild dog.

- Similarly, unless the modern dog owner physically crushes and breaks down the raw vegetable materials fed to modern dogs, those poor animals simply cannot digest them. Not only that, for a dog, they are rarely appetising in "chunky" form.

Why is crushing the vegetables so important ? The answer lies in a bit of elementary high school biology. You will remember that plants, like animals are composed of millions upon millions of cells. The major difference is, plant cells are each surrounded by a cellulose cell wall.

YOUR DOG CANNOT DIGEST CELLULOSE. That means, when you feed lumps of raw carrot or celery, or broccoli, or any type of vegetable to your dog, as so many people do, 99 % of that vegetable material, even if it is very finely grated, is unavailable to your dog. It cannot be digested, and most of it passes straight through, completely unchanged !

- To become available for your dog to use, the contents of each and every cell has to be released from the cellulose cell wall that surrounds it. That means every cell has to be crushed and split open.

Cooking achieves this effect, but at a very high price in terms of lost nutrition. The much preferred way is to physically break the vegetables down without heat as happens in nature when herbivores eat their food.

Your Dog's Raw Veggies Should Resemble the Contents of Sheep's Intestines !

In other words modern dog owners need to mimic that natural process I have just described. Grating is no good because there is no crushing. A food processor does it reasonably well, if you keep it going for long enough, but the most satisfactory way to do it is to put the vegetable material through a juicer.

- You may feed your dog the pulp only and drink the juice yourself, or mix some of the juice back in. People who own [and use] juicers, are learning not to throw the pulp away. Feed that pulp to the dog !

- Another excellent way to crush your vegetables, is to pass them through an old fashioned meat mincer.

Whichever way you do it, the end result is a raw food, a vegetable pulp that your dog easily digests for brilliant, healthy nutrition. This pulp contains fibre, water, minerals [including calcium], enzymes, vitamins, carbohydrates, anti-oxidants, and some proteins and essential fatty acids.

Many clients with bush or farm experience, comment that the texture of this vegetable pulp is similar to the gut contents of sheep, cattle, kangaroos etc.. This is important. Texture, or mouth feel is very important in inducing dogs to eat.

How do You Use It ?

You may feed it to your animal as is. I like to add things to it.

Recipe

- E.g. one of the vegetable oils such as soyabean or safflower oil for energy and more essential fatty acids and anti-oxidants [vitamin E].
- Some brewer's yeast for more B vitamins, including B1 or thiamin, high class protein, selenium, and glucose tolerance factor.
- Some KELP for iodine.. which is deficient in Australian soils.
- A raw egg yolk for extra protein, for choline and more essential fatty acids.
- Some apple cider vinegar, for its acidity and other healthful properties.
- Some yoghurt for the healthy bacteria it contains together with compounds called "pro-biotics" - which promote your dog's health. Pro-biotics can be thought of as acting like natural antibiotics.

WARNING: Do not store this vegetable pulp. It must be fed fresh. It quickly goes off [becomes oxidised], and loses much of it's nutritional value.

What Vegetables Can be Used This Way ?

Present your dog with whatever vegetables are in season. Spinach, broccoli, pumpkin, cabbage, brussel sprouts, cauliflower, green lettuce leaves, red or green peppers, chives, onions, sweet potato, carrots, celery, parsnip, peas, beans... whatever. They are all highly nutritious. The greater the variety the better. You do not even have to spend money. You can buy all the off-cuts from the green grocers, the stuff in the boxes out the back... the stuff they are glad to get rid of for nothing... and feed that to the dogs... suitably processed of course....... RECYCLING WASTE .. PAR EXCELLENCE !

- Note: do not give your dogs excessive amounts of the cabbage family - raw. Large amounts of cabbages, cauliflowers, broccoli and brussel sprouts etc. over a long period, can depress the functioning of the thyroid gland. Similarly, beans and peas should only be fed raw in limited amounts.

I often read or I am told that dogs should not eat raw potatoes. However, many of my clients report their dogs thriving on raw potatoes [suitably crushed], as a regular part of their diet.

- Note that green potatoes are poisonous, to both humans and dogs.

In other words for healthy dogs, all vegetables are fine, with the exceptions I have mentioned, so long as they are properly prepared.

Getting Your Dog to Eat Vegetables

I have not yet found a dog that did not like vegetables when prepared in this manner. Sometimes they needed a bit of hunger as motivation to get them started, but mostly not. It is a very natural, normal food for them, particularly when they are started on it as puppies.

- Always remember that for a dog, the best motivating factor known is hunger.

Several days without food will stimulate a dog's appetite for anything, including vegetables. Particularly if they are prepared correctly. This method is particularly important when you are trying to tempt an over-indulged, obese canine to sample healthier fare.

Many clients over the years have told me in some amazement how their dogs love to eat vegetables. However, most dog owners who have never offered their dog vegetables assume it would be very reluctant to eat them.

In the case of your over-fed, addicted-to-cooked-food dog, I suspect they would be right. Most pampered pooches living in the suburbs would not voluntarily eat vegetables without a motivating factor.

- That is why it is so important to get dogs eating properly from when they are puppies.

However, given the appropriate motivating factors, mainly hunger, practically any dog will grow to love a wide variety of vegetables. You may have to start off with the vegetables lightly steamed. Over a period of time, reduce the proportion of steamed vegetables, so that eventually all of the vegetables are presented as the raw vegetable pulp/mush.

- Note, do not be in a hurry. Make all changes slowly. Sudden changes in diet will sometimes result in upset bowels, colic wind and diarrhoea.

Another very effective motivating factor... for the owner, is when their dog contracts one or more of the degenerative diseases, particularly arthritis. I am always amazed and pleased as people gladly adopt this raw vegetable based diet for their sick dog. The reason they do, is because their beloved pet has been given an agonising death sentence.

It is usually not very long before I see happy clients with a happier, more alive dog. Vegetable based diets work well in alleviating degenerative diseases !

- The bottom line on vegetables, is that your dog needs them, they are best fed raw, and for maximum value to your dog in a nutritional sense, they must be TOTALLY CRUSHED to release their contents. The easiest way to do this is to put them through a juicer and feed the pulp... and as much or as little of the juice as you like.

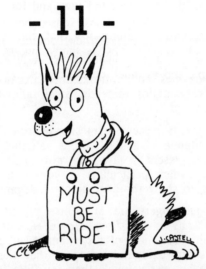

Fruit as Dog Food

Yes, dogs can and do eat fruit. Wild dogs, foxes, dingoes, they all do it. They all eat fruit. Eating fruit is totally natural for dogs. Remember, dogs are omnivores. They can eat anything.

Quite a few clients over the years have told me how their dogs love fruit. I have clients whose dog's fight over fruit in the same way that many dogs fight over bones. Many new clients seem almost afraid or ashamed to tell me their dog eats fruit. It is as if they think I would disapprove. They have this image of vets as only approving of people who feed their dogs commecial dog food. How wrong they are.

So do not be worried if your dog likes fruit. That's great ! Raw fruit is excellent as another nutritious part of your dog's diet. Just as it is for you. Notice I said raw fruit. Cooked fruit, canned fruit, is processed fruit and almost does not count. In common with all other cooked foods, much of it's nutritional value has been lost.

What Nutrients do Dogs get From Raw Fruit ?

Fruits are mostly water. After that, the major nutrient in fruit is soluble carbohydrate. That is simple sugars. Energy foods. Fruit contains lots of fibre, both soluble and insoluble. It also contains vitamins, enzymes and anti-oxidants. Because fruit is a whole food, it also contains minerals, small amounts of protein, and small amounts of fat.

Two nutrients present in most raw fruits, vitamin A as caro-tene, and vitamin C, make fruit a valuable food for your dog. The enzymes present in raw fruit, also make it important as part of your dog's diet, particularly if your dog is past middle age, and starting to show the beginnings of degenerative disease.

The simple sugars are of course present in both raw and cooked fruit, as is the fibre. However, like other foods, once cooked, fruit loses most of it's vitamins, all of it's enzymes and most of it's anti-oxidants. I suspect that the fibre from cooked food is probably less valuable than the fibre from raw foods.

Is it Essential that Dogs Eat Fruit ?

No, definitely not. All of the nutrients present in fruit can be obtained from other sources. However, by adding fruit to your dog's diet, you do one more thing to ensure it is fed on a wide variety of foods. This gives it the greatest chance of receiving a balanced diet with plenty of those longevity and immune system promoting nutrients.

What Fruit Should a Dog Eat ?

That's simple. Any fruit. However, tropical fruits are a parti-cularly valuable food. They contain high levels of enzymes, and lots of anti-oxidants. The cancer free, blemish free skin of dark skinned people living in the hot tropics, owes a lot to a diet chock full of raw tropical fruits. Studies done on these races have shown that when they abandon their traditional diet, and adopt a cooked western diet, their health declines dramatically, with a huge rise in the incidence of degenerative diseases.

Fruit is Youth Food

The modern scientific study of life extension is revealing why fruit is such a valuable food. Why it is able to keep humans and animals, youthful in mind and body into advanced age.

Scientists have discovered that between them, the enzymes and the anti-oxidants present in fruit, many of which have not yet been identified, keep the skin and indeed the whole body free of degeneration and old age diseases. One of the ways fruit does this is to reduce cross linking, a major cause of ageing.

The older the dog, the more important it is that fruit form a part of it's diet. Fruit is youth food for your dog. It is particularly valuable for arthritic dogs. Another reason that fruit is youth food, is because it is low in fat and low in protein.

Whole ? Green ? Ripe ? Over-Ripe ?

Which is best ? In nature, the dog being a scavenger, browses on fruit that has fallen from trees, or gulps down half-digested fruit from the belly of it's prey. In other words dogs require to eat very ripe to over-ripe fruit..... raw of course !

The over-ripe fruit, unlike green fruit, will not cause digestive upsets. Instead it will contain maximum levels of simple sugars, valuable fibre, particularly the soluble kind, vitamins, enzymes, and anti-oxidants.

Really rotten fruit should not be fed. It may produce botulism in your dog. This is a disease caused by bacteria which paralyses your dog and can kill it.

If the fruit you have is not fully ripe, either let it ripen, or if it is ripe but firm, put it through the juicer and feed it to your dog that way. Once again, like feeding vegetables to your dog, with under-ripe fruit, you are battling cellulose cell walls.

To release each cell's contents for your dog to digest, you need to somehow physically break down the cells... and the juicer is the best way I know of doing it. [see feeding vegetables .. previous chapter.]

Fruit can be fed at any time. We tend to feed fruit by itself, either as a large meal of fruit, or as snacks, or before other food.

If a dog has not eaten fruit before, you may need to use a little bit of hunger to induce him or her to start. Alternatively, mix some in with what your dog will eat, and gradually increase the amount of fruit offered in that mix.

What About Dried Fruit ?

Dried fruits, particularly sun dried fruits are an excellent addition to the canine diet. Apart from their intrinsic food value, they are an excellent natural laxative, which can be valuable when large amounts of bones have been eaten for example.

Both raisins and sultanas, but partuicularly raisins are an good source of iron. This is important for those folk who prefer not to feed their dogs any animal products.

Honey as Dog Food

Honey as raw food for dogs is excellent. Unfortunately, ninety nine percent of the honey in shops, and this includes a lot of so called health food shops has been heat extracted as opposed to cold extracted. This means that once again, many of the health promoting attributes have been killed, making it basically just one more source of soluble carbohydrates. However, even in the heat extracted form, it is still far more nutritious than straight sugar or straight glucose, and less likely to be a cause of sugar diabetes. This is because of the types of sugars it contains.

Honey is an excellent source of instant energy for mothers, sick dogs, young dogs, old dogs, in diabetic crises etc.

- Note that in general, soluble carbohydrates are not good foods for racing or hard working animals, immediately prior to the exercise bout.

Raw honey, in common with other raw foods contains many more health giving nutrients than cooked honey. This includes enzymes and B vitamins.

For humans, and one would therefore assume for dogs, there will be the occasional individual who is allergic to the pollens in raw honey.

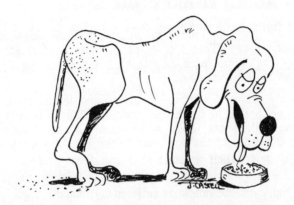

Grains and Legumes as Dog Food

I have grouped grains and legumes together for a number of reasons. Firstly, they are both seed type foods. Secondly, being seeds, they both require to be cooked. Thirdly, when feeding them to dogs, it is better if they are fed together.

They should be fed together because in a number of ways, each contains what the other lacks. Grains lack the amino acid Lysine and legumes lack the amino acid methionine. Grains are high in phosphorus and low in calcium, while legumes are high in calcium.

By combining these two foods in approximately equal amounts ... at the same meal, you will be producing a food which is correctly balanced for both amino acids and also for calcium and phosphorus. For example, instead of feeding just rice to your dog, add some type of legume. It can be as simple as a can of baked beans.

However, do not be mislead. None of this means I strongly recommend either of them as dog food. I give you this information as an indication of how best to use them, and particularly because so many people use one of these foods when feeding their dogs, but not the other.

Commonly, dog owners feed grains without legumes. That is fine in small amounts. However, what is not fine, is when either grains or legumes become a major part of their dog's diet as is so common today. That sort of eating may be OK for humans [although that is not necesarily true], but it is not for dogs. That brings me to the next point.

Another reason for grouping grains and legumes together, is because neither is to be recommended in large amounts as food for dogs. Neither are foods which have figured prominently in the eating history of the dog prior to the last fifty years or so.

- There is much circumstantial and direct evidence linking the consumption of both of them in large amounts to many disease problems suffered by modern dogs.

LEGUMES AS DOG FOOD

Apart from sprouted legumes, and fresh vegetables such as peas and beans, the legumes I refer to here are the dry seeds. As such they have to be either soaked or cooked or both, before you can feed them to your dog.

As I have mentioned, combined with grains in about equal amounts, they are useful as dog food. However, they are cooked, they have to be, so this immediately reduces their nutritional value, and is a major reason I recommend against using large amounts of them.

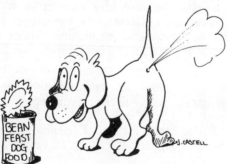

Apart from that, they contain high levels of starch, moderate levels of reasonable to poor protein, and they are capable of generating in your dog, a lot of "wind". This is a definite problem in deep chested dogs which are inclined to "bloat".

Legumes do not usually cause a problem if they are only a small part of a dog's diet. Unfortunately, many home cooked recipes for dogs and quite a few commercial dog foods contain high levels of legumes, eg. soyabean meal. This is not good nutrition for a dog. The results obtained when dogs are fed these sorts of diets for any extended period of time bear witness to this.

WARNING: Many commercial dog foods full of lovely look-ing chunky meaty pieces, do not contain meat. That supposed meat, which looks as though it has been carved directly off a big lump of steak, is in fact textured vegetable protein. Pure soy protein. With all the inherent problems of cooked protein from legumes.

- The bottom line is that cooked legumes are fine in small amounts as a minor component in your dog's diet. A diet that should be based on raw meaty bones. They are not however, recommended as a major part of a dog's diet.

GRAIN AS DOG FOOD

Grain, particularly cooked grain is not a food the dog has evolved to eat in large quantities, and yet that is precisely what a lot of modern folk ask their dog to exist on.

Most domestic dogs eat a diet based largely on grain. This is because they eat commercial dog food, and most commercial dog foods have a high grain component. This includes most canned and soft moist dog foods and practically all dry dog foods.

Commercial dog foods are based on grain because it is cheap and available. Certainly not because it is the best food to feed dogs.

Another group that regularly feed grains to their dogs are the health food faddists. Usually people who follow the "Macrobiotic ideas" or the "Pritikin-type" diets. These people tend to feed their dogs the same way they feed themselves. They use rice, usually brown, but sometimes white, as the basis of the diet.

This is done very much for economic reasons, and partly because they have faith in such diets.

- Unfortunately, grain based diets are implicated in all sorts of allergies and other health problems such as arthritis and cancer in human beings.

One culprit is the protein called gluten found in grain, particularly wheat. That is why so called health foods often boast of being "gluten free". However, grain problems go much deeper than that.

A fundamental problem for humans is, they have only been eating grain in large quantities for about 10,000 years. That is, in many respects, it is still an unnatural food for us. Our internal make up is still not designed by long evolution to cope with loads of grain. We are better adapted to eating fruit, vegetables and to a lesser extent meat.

The dog is in exactly the same position, only more so. Whereas humans have had about 10,000 years to get used to eating cooked grains, most breeds of dogs have only been fed cooked grain in any quantity for between 30 and 100 years. There may be the odd breed round the world which has been kept on a basically grain diet for longer, but that would not be common. In fact, for the majority of Aussie dogs, copious grain eating has only been going on for about 30 years. That is, since the introduction of commercial dog foods on a large scale in Australia, particularly dry dog foods, in 1966.

Grain feeding does not usually cause immediate problems. Dogs are scavengers and omnivores which means they can cope with just about any food, cooked or raw without problems.. for short periods or in small amounts.

- It is when a generally unsuitable food, such as grain, is fed as most of the diet for a number of years that problems begin to surface.

Dogs that eat grain as the major part of their diet suffer premature ageing and the early development of degenerative diseases, such as arthritis, cancer, diabetes, and other pancreatic problems. Many skin problems, allergic problems and arthritic problems respond to the withdrawl of grains from a dog's diet.

Why do Grain Based Diets Cause Problems ?

They are a Cooked Food

Grains have to be cooked because dogs cannot digest them raw. Grains contain enzyme inhibitors. Cooking destroys those enzyme inhibitors allowing dog's to digest them.

- The problems with cooked food have been discussed at length. You will remember they include losses of vitamins, fibre, enzymes, anti-oxidants and other longevity/health factors. In other words, lost nutritional value. Loss of health promoting power.

Full of Soluble Carbohydrates

When a dog eats any grain based product, for example bread, dry dog food, a' rice based home made diet etc., it is receiving a product containing about 70 % carbohydrate. Most of this is starch with a little bit of fibre.

- Unfortunately, starch, once cooked, has a reaction in the body not much different to feeding pure sugar.

That is, such products fed over a long period of time are likely to cause any disease which can be attributed to a diet high in soluble carbohydrates... particularly sugar diabetes. This is particularly true of breads, especially white breads. Of the grains, it is the very popular rice which acts most like sugar.

Grains Cause Mineral Imbalances

Grains fed in large amounts without legumes, cause problems because they are unbalanced nutritionally with respect to a dog's mineral needs.

- They are high in phosphorus and low in calcium. That low calcium is not good for the bones of dogs of any age, but is particularly bad for the bones of growing pups. The high phosphorus is not good for the kidneys of adult dogs.

Grains Contain Small Amounts of Poor Quality Protein

In general, the protein quality of grains should be regarded as poor and not easily available to your dog. Grains are deficient in the amino acid lysine, and compared to animal proteins, plant proteins are poorly digested.

The protein content in grain varies quite a bit. It ranges from about 6 or 7 % in rice, up to about 17 % in some wheats.

Most grains average about 12 % protein. This is too low for a growing pup. It would be quite a reasonable level for an adult dog if it was good quality protein, but as I have mentioned it is not.

- Unfortunately, rice, the most popular of the grains that people feed to their dogs, is the one with the lowest levels of protein, and possibly the poorest quality protein.

Grains Actively Stop the Absorption of Calcium

They do this in two ways. Firstly because they lack the amino acid lysine, and secondly because they contain phosphorous compounds called "phytates".

Your dog's body requires the amino acid lysine [the one missing from grains] as a carrier for calcium. Lysine ensures that enough calcium is absorbed from the gut and distributed to where it is needed.

The compounds in grains called phytates tend to bind Calcium. This makes the already low levels of calcium in cereals even more unavailable. The low lysine further ensures that not much calcium is absorbed. This makes a mostly cereal diet a pretty calcium deficient diet.... not much good for a growing pup. Not much good for a growing pup's bones. Not good for an adult dog on a low calcium diet.

Those phytates also bind other essential minerals such as zinc and chromium and selenium, making them unavailable to your dog as well.

Grains are Very Poor Food for Growing Pups

- If cereals are fed in large amounts to growing dogs, it is important to make sure that plenty of bones are being fed at the same time.

The first reason for this is the low calcium [and other minerals] levels in cereals as just described. The second reason is because lysine, the amino acid missing from cereals is a key amino acid in the formation of collagen, which is the major protein in bone, cartilage and conective tissue, including skin.

Bones make up for this deficiency. Another factor involved here is the lack of vitamin C in a diet based largely on grain. Vitamin C is an essential nutrient in collagen and therefore bone and other tissue formation.

- As mentioned, grain based diets are low in zinc which is essential for skin health, bone growth and general growth, for immune system health, for proper development of the organs of reproduction and so on.

With respect to fat content and essential fatty acids, most whole grains contain no more than 2 % fat and more is needed for dogs, especially for growing dogs. The exception to this is oats with 7 % fat.

- It does not take a lot of imagination to realise that a diet high in cereals, with not much else added, which is commonly fed to both adults and growing pups, is bound to cause bone and other growth problems.

Grain Based Diets are Poor Skin Food.

A predominantly cereal diet [EG. MOST COMMERCIAL DOG FOODS] is a great recipe for skin disaster. Collagen, the basic framework on which skin is built is formed poorly on a grain based diet. Many nutrients are necessary for the production of healthy skin. These include, amongst others, good quality protein with plenty of lysine, vitamin C, essential fatty acids, the B complex including biotin, and zinc. All of these are poorly available from a predominantly grain diet.

Modern dogs are plagued with skin problems. Most animal health care professionals are kept busy, particularly in the warmer months treating these very preventable conditions. The occasional thought may be given to a "wheat allergy" and on that basis it may be suggested that grains be withdrawn from the diet.

In a small percentage of cases, a simple allergy may be the problem. However, the vast majority of skin conditions are built on nothing less than a totally unsuitable diet. That is, a grain based diet. In other words, the resulting skin problems are due to a much wider range of problems than a simple allergy. They are caused by a wide range of nutritional deficiencies and imbalances.

- Unfortunately, once these conditions are set in motion, and have been present for a number of years, they are almost impossible to treat successfully. Even with a proper diet !

They will improve vastly, but the dogs often have to spend the rest of their lives being medicated, because the original nutritional insult, that largely grain based diet, leaves their body permanently damaged.

Grains and Allergies

Most allergies are developed because unsuitable foods are introduced to puppies at too young an age. Instead of leaving pups on mother's milk [often because mother can not make sufficient milk for long enough because of poor modern feeding habits - i.e. commercial dog food], pups are weaned early.

- Commonly, as with humans, they will be weaned on to some grain based cereal.

This is a widespread and much applauded practice, and yet is not to be recommended. It is a great recipe for sensitising the young pup's body to wheat protein, and setting it up for allergies later on in life. Much better to feed mum properly on bone based diets, so that she is able to produce sufficient healthy milk for her pups until they are at least five or preferably six weeks old, and then gradually wean the pups using raw meaty bone mince.

Grains ... Not a Great Idea for Dogs

In other words the majority of dogs, that is, all the dogs eating grain based commercial dog food, are being fed a food for which their physiology [their internal workings] is totally unsuited.

Let us now examine the common grains that are fed to dogs, looking at their individual characteristics as they relate to a dog's nutrition and health.

Rice as Dog Food

This is without doubt one of the most popular bases for home produced dog foods. This popularity is partly for economic reasons .... the stuff is really cheap, and partly on supposed health grounds.... The belief that a healthy diet is being produced.

- Rice is great invalid food. This is because it is easily digested. It does not place any great strain on an already taxed system, and it has useful properties which help resolve health problems involving diarrhoea.

Rice, particularly white rice, is almost pure starch. Instant energy. Low in protein of poor quality. It's protein is deficient in lysine. This is not a problem if rice is fed in small amounts or for short periods, or if it is sensibly combined with other foods to make up for it's shortcomings.

- However, if rice is fed over a lifetime, as the basis of the whole diet, particularly if it is white rice, several nutritional errors are likely to be made... depending on how much rice is fed, and what other foods are added to the mix.

The first error, particularly with white rice, is a diet very high in what is almost a soluble carbohydrate. Research has shown, and clinical experience bears this out.

- I have seen many instances of dogs fed copious quantities of rice, and in many instances it was brown rice, all their lives end up with pancreatic disease, which includes diabetes, Pancreatic Insufficiency, and Pancreatitis.

The second problem, is a diet which does not have enough total protein, and a diet deficient in one particular essential amino acid.. lysine.

The third error, particularly if white rice is used, is a diet low in fibre.

At this stage you could be forgiven for thinking that I am telling you not to feed rice to your dog. Not at all. Do it. After all, the Orientals have been eating it for thousands of years very succesfully.

- The trick is to use smaller amounts of it together with other foods. Foods which will make up for it's deficiencies. Use it in such a way as it will produce a healthy dog.

The most important food is of course RAW MEATY BONES such as chicken wings or meaty lamb off cuts, or scraps of pork on the bone. They add essential fatty acids, they balance up the protein, and instantly fix the lack of minerals, particularly calcium and zinc. However, I get ahead of myself here, practical feeding comes in the next section.

Wheat as Dog Food

All the general comments I made about grains apply very much to wheat. Compared to rice, wheat is actually quite a nutritious grain. It has about twice as much protein, more fibre, higher in vitamin E content, and is high in some of the B vitamins. Because it contains the protein gluten, it is used to make bread. The gluten is what holds the little gas bubbles.... allowing the bread to rise.

Nobody that I know of, goes out and buys wheat to feed their dogs. Not the way they do with rice for example. However, plenty of wheat products are fed to dogs, the most common in Australia being commercial dog food, with dry dog food having the highest content of wheat and other grains.

Some farmers will take wheat based stock foods and feed it to their dogs. When combined with meat meal and raw meaty bones, together with lots of cattle, and/or sheep and/or horse faeces, and possibly vegetable scraps, these dogs will do quite well.

The other very common wheat products people feed their dogs is pasta and bread. Well, that is fine, in small amounts. I have already mentioned that bread, especially white bread in large amounts will have much the same effect on your dog as feeding pure sugar... so do not do it !

A lot of people feed young puppies a diet consisting mainly of a human breakfast cereals made from wheat. All the comments I made about grain and the problems it causes with growth, and in particular, growing bones applies here. These human cereals are particularly bad because of the added sugar.

- You must let raw meaty bones form the bulk of a puppy's diet if it is to be healthy and have healthy bones.

Oats as Dog Food

If you really want to feed grain products to your dog.... think strongly about feeding oats. Rolled oats. Of the grains, oats is about the best grain for your dog.

- Rolled oats have the highest fat levels of all the grains, a whopping great 7 or 8 %, and that fat is high in essential fatty acids.
- Oats are high in protein. They have 15 % which is two and a half times more protein than rice.
- Oats are a good source of minerals. They have the highest calcium of all the grains [twice as much as rice], and good levels of iron, zinc, potassium, and manganese.
- Oats have good levels of vitamin E and the B vitamins. Oats have much higher levels of dietary fibre than other grains, much of it being the valuable soluble type.

However, before you get too excited, when you buy rolled oats, you buy a heat treated product. It has been passed through heated rollers, a process which is necessary to destroy the enzyme inhibitors. Also remember, it is still a grain, which means it's protein is deficient in lysine. In other words, despite those good things you have just read, it can only form part of your dog's diet, and should not form the bulk of it.

Some people tell me of stories they have read about working dogs in Scotland existing and being very healthy on a diet consisting almost solely of oats.

Oats may have made up the bulk of their diet, but they were probably also given unpasteurised milk and possibly eggs. In addition, those dogs would have consumed many other "foods". Their diet would have included faeces, soil, many different grasses and herbs, small animals such as rats and mice together with the carcases of dead sheep.

- They balanced their own diets on a whole lot more than oats !

Other Grains .. E.g. Corn, Rye, Millet, Barley etc.

Since these are not readily available in large amounts, there is no real point in pursuing their individual attributes as food for your dog. No doubt each has its own particular values and characteristics. The best approach to adopt here, is, if you want to feed these foods to your dog, do so, in small amounts, occasionally, as part of a VARIED diet and if possible, balanced by a legume.

- In other words, feed NOTHING EXCLUSIVELY to your dog. Most particularly do not base your dog's diet on grain. Base it on raw meaty bones, preferably chicken pieces.

Bread as Dog Food.

Bread is usually made from flour, gluten [a protein], yeast, oil, salt, with various chemicals added such as emulsifiers and preservatives.

As a food for dogs it is unbalanced, particularly with regard to the essential amino acids. The carbohydrate part, the starch or the flour, particularly in a white loaf is not dissimilar to pure sugar in it's effects on your dog's body, although whole meal bread is a lot better in this respect. It is not high in essential fatty acids. It does supply energy, but mostly from soluble carbohydrates. The salt part will not do a lot of harm unless other foods with excess salt, such as commercial dog foods, make up most of the diet. Basically, it is devoid of most vitamins, most minerals, and is particularly low in calcium.

If you are feeding bread, feed it in small amounts only as part of a broadly based diet.

Sprouted Grain

This is a very healthy and natural way to feed grain to your dog. It is a way of feeding grain without cooking it. That means your dog obtains all the benefits of the whole raw grain with none of the draw backs. In fact, once the sprouting process has begun, that grain is a power pack of nutrition. Much more valuable than the dormant seed nutritionally.

- This is because the newly sprouted seed contains all of the original nutrients plus an incredible increase in the vitamin content, including the vitamins A, B complex, C and E.

If you wish to feed sprouted grain to your dog, pop along to your local health food store where they will be pleased to supply you with both the grain and detailed instructions for getting started.

IMPORTANT: Do make sure the grain is food grain. Do not use seed grain. Most seed grain has been treated chemically and is poisonous.

Briefly, all you require is a glass jar, lots of clean running water, the grain, a piece of cloth to put over the top of the jar and a rubber band to keep the cloth in place. I use wheat as the grain, it is readily available, cheap, and sprouts with reasonable ease. Note that grain takes longer to sprout than legumes.

Soak the grain for about twenty four to forty eight hours in water. Change the water twice daily while it is soaking. When the grains are obviously swollen, tip the water out, rinse well several times, cover the top of the jar with the cloth, and lay the glass jar on its side with the bottom end slightly elevated so that any water drains out.

Keep the grain in the dark during the soaking and sprouting.

Again, rinse the grain several times a day during this period. Once the grain begins to sprout, spread it out thinly in the sun on absorbent paper until the shoots turn green, or alternatively, just place the whole jar out in the sun, and keep moving the grains and rinsing them [24 to 48 hours]. Now it is ready to use.

IMPORTANT: Do not allow big long shoots to form, you want it just sprouted and that is all. Use it as you would any other vegetable material, by crushing and grinding it. Use it immediately after that process. Store excess uncrushed grain in the refrigerator as you would any other sprouted seed.

It is not necessary to use this sprouted grain in enormous quantities. Mix a handful or two with other vegetable material.

- Sprouted grain is the MOST healthy way to feed grain to your dog, and once crushed, very closely mimics the stomach contents of a grazing animal. It is a top quality product which will contribute enormously to your dog's health and wellbeing. If you have the time to prepare it, I cannot recommend it too strongly.

Sprouted Legumes

These will sprout more quickly than grains. In general, follow the advice as given for grains, except halve the time for soaking, and just leave the sprouting seeds in the jar when you pop them out in the sun to green up.

Like the grains, they should be eaten when they have just sprouted. This is when their nutritional value is maximal. If you allow them to grow long and leggy as they are in the shops, much of their nutritional value has been lost.

Incidentally, with experience, you will find your own unique method of sprouting seeds, the one that works best for you.

- 13 -

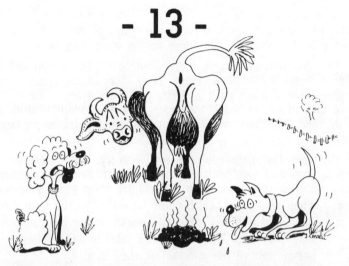

Dairy Products as Food for Your Dog

Modern dairy products are not entirely health promoting. This is because they are not raw....They have been pasteurised ... cooked. In common with all cooked foods, they do not usually cause immediate problems. They simply do not promote long term health.

- Pasteurisation, destroys B vitamins, vitamin C, anti-oxidants, enzymes and other longevity and health promoting factors found in raw milk. In addition it denatures the proteins, making them less useful, and sometimes indigestible.

A further problem occurs when milk is homogenised. The process releases a chemical which damages the inside walls of blood vessels, thus contributing to cardiovascular disease.

Raw Milk Promotes Health

A recent study of the health of dairy farmers and their families, who ate and drank copious quantities of raw milk, and raw milk products, showed that these people were very healthy.

One hundred years ago, there were health farms that fed their clients nothing but raw milk. They very successfully treated degenerative disease such as arthritis, heart disease, kidney disease and so on, in much the same way as modern health farms with their emphasis on raw fruit and vegetables enjoy similar success.

Compare that to a couple I met recently. They were in their fifties, both had had heart attacks and both had developed crippling arthritis since moving to the country three years previously.

- Their decline in health could be traced to the time they purchased a Jersey cow, and began to use her produce in vast quantities. They made one fatal mistake. They pasteurised all the milk before they used it.

Milk is pasteurised to prevent the transmission of Tuberculosis and other disease problems from cows to people. Those reasons are valid when milk is being produced under diverse conditions for large numbers of people and needs to be transported, stored and guaranteed as "pure".

On a farm, where hygiene can be controlled and a cow can be checked for the absence of such diseases, pasteurisation is unnecesary, and positively harmful.

Despite all that, pasteurised milk products can be used as part of a balanced healthy diet for our omnivorous, scavenging friend the dog.

- However, milk and it's products are not an essential part of a dog's diet. The nutrients in milk are just as easily provided by other foods such as raw meaty bones, green veggies and liver or cod liver oil for example.

Cows Milk as Dog Food

Milk is the most common dairy product fed to dogs, especially to young puppies. Milk provides water,calcium, magnesium,

sodium and potassium, very little iron or zinc, good quality protein, saturated fat, some vitamin A and traces of the B vitamins.

However, as I have mentioned, feeding pasteurised milk to
your dog is about as good as feeding any other cooked food. On
the other hand, if you can get hold of raw milk from a certified
disease free cow, then what you are feeding is a whole lot better. In fact just about a complete food.

- Apart from the fact that it is cooked, the main problem
  with milk is that it will cause in susceptible individuals,
  tummy upsets, skin problems and diarrhoea.

The diarrhoea is very common, particularly with young pups.
There are three reasons that diarrhoea occurs. Two uncommon,
and one very common. Fortunately, the common one can be
avoided by suitably modifying the milk. Not only that, the modi-
fied milk is much more nutritious for your dog.

Milk, Allergies - and Diarrhoea

Milk can cause diarrhoea, skin problems, rhinitis, or even lung
problems due to an allergic reaction to one or more of it's proteins. However, these are not all that common in dogs. The most
likely candidate would be a teenage or adult dog fed cow's milk
as a very young puppy.

Allergies to cow's milk are avoided by not feeding it or foods
that contain it. That usually means eliminating processed foods
from your dog's diet. Many of them contain milk by-products.

- As I routinely advise elimination of commercial dog foods
  from the diets of dogs in general, and sickly dogs in
  particular, all those allergic problems are usually
  eliminated anyway.

Intolerance to Milk Sugar - and Diarrhoea

Some dogs develop a frothy smelly diarrhoea when they drink
cow's milk. The cause is an inability to digest the milk sugar or
lactose.

- This occurs because some dogs, particularly after they are weaned, do not produce the enzyme lactase which is required for digesting lactose.

Instead of the milk sugar being broken down into simple sugars and absorbed, it is attacked by bacteria which convert it to volatile fatty acids plus the gases hydrogen and carbon dioxide. The bowel contents become extremely acid. This irritates the bowel and prevents water re-absorption. The net result is frothy, smelly diarrhoea.

- The problem is overcome by either not feeding cow's milk or by feeding the dog yoghurt, which does not contain lactose, or by feeding watered-down cow's milk.

Soy milk does not have lactose, however, it does have it's problems and I shall discuss those shortly.

Some lactose intolerant dogs and pups can drink goat's milk without problems. This may be because it is raw, and still contains it's own enzymes.

Another alternative is to use one of the synthetic low lactose milks currently available today. Either from your vet or from supermarkets, chemists etc..

Cow's Milk, Low Nutrient Value - and Diarrhoea

Until recently it was believed that lactose intolerance as I have just described, was the main reason for dogs getting diarrhoea when they drank cow's milk.

Part of the problem was supposed to be due to the higher levels of lactose in cow's milk. In fact, both bitch's and cow's have approximately equal concentrations of lactose in their milk.

- Most of the diarrhoea seen when dogs drink milk is related to another difference between bitch's and cow's milk.

Bitch's milk is twice as concentrated as cow's milk. It has twice as much energy, protein and fat as cows milk, but the same amount of lactose.

Recent experiments with greyhounds which developed diarrhoea whenever they drank cow's milk, showed that when fed cow's milk fortified with whey protein and canola oil, the dogs produced normal stools with no sign of diarrhoea. Just why the improvement occurs is not precisely clear. It has to do with higher energy levels, higher protein levels and the dilution of lactose. The important thing is the results..... no diarrhoea !

This ties in with observations made by many breeders world wide, myself included, that when sufficient egg yolks are added to cow's milk [egg yolks being rich in both fats and protein], bitches, puppies and convalescing dogs in general do very well and do not get diarrhoea. .

Safe Milk for Dogs - Recipe

- The mix I use is a cup of milk [250 ml], plus 2 egg yolks, one or two teaspoons of canola oil, a teaspoon of honey, and a small pinch of salt. This particular mixture works very well as a stimulant to milk production in bitches unable to supply enough milk to a litter of puppies.
- Another use for that mix is as an excellent emergency substitute milk for orphan pups. To improve it for those pups, add a few drops of a complete vitamin supplement. One containing all the B vitamins, vitamin C, and vitamins A, D, E and K.

Do note that this mix, if given to a very young puppy can result in allergies to egg protein later on in life. However, better that than dead pups.

New Milk Product for Puppies

- If you think your puppies may require supplementary feeding, there is a new product called "Biolac". Ask your vet about it. It has produced excellent results in orphan puppies.

A common method used to allow dogs with "apparent lactose intolerance" to drink milk, has been to drastically dilute it, and then gradually strengthen it, backing off as soon as diarrhoea occurred.

In the light of current evidence, it would appear far more sensible to adopt the increase in total solids approach. Note that this cannot be done in the case of a true milk allergy, or a true lactose intolerance.

- The only way you can find out if your dog can tolerate this fortified milk mix is to .... feed it !

Goats Milk

Goat's milk is a highly nutritious food. One of it's greatest benefits is that it is available RAW. That means all the health promoting factors of enzymes, anti-oxidants and other longevity factors are still present.

The composition of cow's milk and goat's milk is roughly equivalent, except that goat's milk has more sodium and more potassium, and less calcium, protein and fat than cow's milk. Like cow's milk it is low in the minerals zinc and iron, but has good quantities of magnesium. It seems less able to cause allergies than cow's milk.

Raw goat's milk has proved itself useful as a milk substitute for young puppies. Why it has less problems in this respect than cow's milk is not totally clear. However, goat's milk is more easily digested, particularly by young animals. This is because it produces a more alkaline reaction in the stomach, and, compared to cow's milk, forms a soft, friable, much more easily digested curd. It may also be because goat's milk has a more favourable fatty acid balance. The fat is more digestible. The globules are finer and goat's milk is naturally homogenised.

- Obviously, goat's milk as a substitute for bitch's milk would be a better product with the addition of egg yolks, canola oil and B vitamins or brewer's yeast.

On the down side, goat's milk contains no Beta carotene. This means it cannot contribute any vitamin A to the animal consuming it.

Another problem with goat's milk is very low levels of the vitamins folic acid, and vitamin B6. This would only be a problem where no other foods were being fed. Folic acid is found in poultry, eggs, and green leafy vegetables. B6 is found in fish, legumes, pork, poultry and other meats. So long as these foods are not over processed, these vitamins will be available.

With adult dogs, so long as goat's milk, is not the major part of their diet, so long as the dog is not allergic to it and does not get diarrhoea when given it, then no problems... go right ahead and feed it. A valuable RAW food for your dog. Remember, adding egg yolks, canola oil and brewer's yeast will make this an excellent healthy drink for your dog.

Soy Milk

I include soy milk at this point because so many people want to use it as a substitute for cow's milk. My strong advice is .. don't.

- It is poorly digested, has a poor amino acid profile and the phytates in it tend to bind the calcium. It really is not a worthwhile food for your dog.
- If you must feed it, you would have to add egg and calcium to make it at all worthwhile.

Cheese

Cheese is dried out milk. As dog food, it is a source of protein and fat. It is of course a cooked food. It has had the whey removed which includes the milk sugar lactose, and the amino acid taurine.

It is obviously not a complete food. However, as PART of a varied diet, feeding cheese in small amounts to your dog is fine. Just do not go overboard and let your dog train you to feed it cheese all the time. Lots of cheese will result in excesses of protein, calcium, salt and fat, to the detriment of your dog's health. Many small dogs train their owners to do just that.

Because it has had the lactose or milk sugar removed, it may safely be fed to dogs with a lactose intolerance. [See above.] However, the calcium present in it will not be as well absorbed as the calcium present in milk because of the absence of lactose.

Lactose is important in calcium absorption. The quality of the protein in cheese is high, but cheese is low in essential fatty acids.

- Cheese is definitely not a food you would feed to an old dog with a heart problem because of the high sodium content.

Cottage Cheese

This is great food for your dog. For your dog of any age, from puppies through to geriatric dogs. From sick dogs to totally well dogs. It's greatest feature is that the protein present is highly digestible and of top quality.

The protein in cottage cheese contains high levels of what are called branch chain amino acids. These are a group of three essential amino acids [Leucine, Isoleucine and Valine] which aid wound healing, and help build up muscle. That is why cottage cheese is a valuable food for dogs recovering from any sort of illness. It is also excellent food for growing puppies, for pregnant bitches, for lactating bitches and for dogs that work hard ... athletes.

- This is a food to keep in mind whenever you want to supplement a dog's diet with a cheap, growth promoting, easily digestible, high quality protein.

You would not feed cottage cheese in large amounts to a dog with severe heart problems. It has moderately high levels of sodium. Although it does not have such high levels as ordinary cheese, it does have twice as much sodium as potassium. Of the various types of cottage cheese available the worst one in this respect is creamed low fat cottage cheese which has twice as much sodium as the others.

Yoghurt

Plain yoghurt with the living culture present is an excellent food for dogs. This is because it is a live food. In many ways it is like one of the wild dogs' natural foods, faces, which also derives its principal food value from the fact that it is full of living [and dead] bacteria.

- Basically it is milk that has had the milk sugar in it converted to lactic acid by a bacterial culture. It is the presence of this bacterial culture that gives yoghurt some of its most important health giving properties for your dog.

Yoghurt is an excellent source of calcium, high class protein, vitamins including the B vitamins and vitamin A [no vitamin C], enzymes and of course energy as carbohydrates, protein and fat. It is not a good source of essential fatty acids, and has similar cholesterol levels to milk.

The bacteria present in yoghurt are friendly bacteria. They will live happily in your dog's bowels, as part of your dog's normal bowel flora. In this role it is assumed they will produce more of their probiotics, enzymes, high class proteins, essential fatty acids, vitamins [including vitamin K] etc., which will have the effect of keeping the bowel itself healthy on a local level, and also, many of their health giving products will be absorbed into the rest of the body.

- Yoghurt can be added to ANY dog's food, sick or well. It is of great benefit to young puppies, including orphan puppies, as part of their milk formula.

Yoghurt can be of great benefit when a dog has diarrhoea, particularly when it is suspected that the normal friendly bacteria of the gut have disappeared and been replaced by unfriendly pathogenic bacteria, or where the balance of bacteria in the gut have been upset by the use of broad spectrum antibiotics.

In other words yoghurt can be used to normalise the bacteria in your dog's bowel. The mechanism is not entirely clear. However, it is partly because the bacteria in yoghurt produce substances called probiotics.... rather like natural antibiotics.

Whether the bacteria in the yoghurt are actually able to re-establish the normal flora of the bowel is not entirely certain. Whatever the mechanism, yoghurt is without doubt of benefit in this situation.

If your dog has to take antibiotics, feed it yoghurt. The yoghurt protects against the killing effect that antibiotics have on the normal bowel bacteria. This is particularly useful if antibiotics cause your dog to develop diarrhoea.

Let me also say that yoghurt as part of a varied diet is of great nutritional benefit to your dog.

One more thing...... you do not have to feed your dog the unhealthy sugar filled variety. Use natural yoghurt.

BUTTER AND CREAM

These are pure fat. They are great energy foods. They are high in saturated fatty acids, salt and cholesterol. They do not contain any of the essential fatty acids. They are also high in vitamin A. Small amounts are fine in the diet of a healthy dog.

If they are made from raw milk, they have all the health giving properties of any other raw food.

Margarine - Don't Buy It - Don't Use It !

This is a dairy food substitute made from plant oils. It was advocated in the 1950's for human heart patients because it is capable of blocking the synthesis of cholesterol in humans and presumably in other animals as well.

The problems with this approach to disease prevention could fill their own chapter. Margarine is a totally artificial food for which no currently alive animal [including dogs and humans] is suited. The bottom line is that the extensive use of margarine is linked with cancer, but unfortunately, not with any lessening of coronary heart disease.

In other words margarine is definitely NOT a health food. If you must have it in the house, be kind to your dog and make sure he or she does not get any.

- 14 -

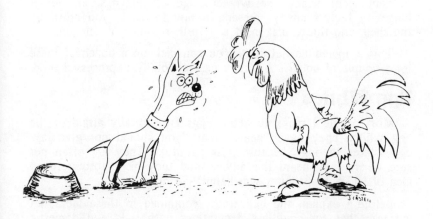

Eggs as Dog Food

I am constantly amazed by people who buy expensive poor quality pet foods for their animals, when there are cheap highly nutritious foods available.

Nothing illustrates this point more than the humble egg. Eggs are dirt cheap, but they are absolutely brilliant nutrition for your dog.

- They are one of the cheapest sources of high quality protein and essential fatty acids you can buy. Eggs are a whole food. They contain all the nutrients required for the growth of a new chicken. Not only that, eggs are always available, and they come completely unprocessed... raw.

The egg is regarded as having the perfect protein. It is the one against which all other proteins are measured. It contains a full complement of minerals, including excellent levels of calcium [mostly in the yolk], all the vitamins except vitamin C and a range of high quality saturated and unsaturated fatty acids, the nutrient lecithin and the whole range of enzymes and other longevity factors always present in raw foods. If you crush up the shell, and throw that in, it is a further source of calcium.

This is incredible nutrition. You can pick up a dozen of these for a couple of dollars. A totally natural totally unprocessed food.

Egg Whites

Most people I speak to about eggs are mortally afraid of the egg white. They have "heard" that "you should not give raw egg whites to dogs, because it is harmful." They are often not sure where they heard this advice, and they have absolutely no idea of HOW egg whites will harm their dog.

Before I explain the half truths contained in these ideas, let me say, that for countless generations both wild and domestic dogs have consumed egg whites, RAW, along with the yolks when robbing birds' nests and stealing eggs. This has caused no problems. No harm whatsoever has occurred. My dogs regularly receive whole raw eggs as part of a balanced natural diet. No problems. Just the opposite. Brilliant health.

So what is all the fuss about ?

EGG WHITES HAVE TWO PROBLEMS
- Firstly they contain an ENZYME INHIBITOR which can make them difficult to digest for a very young puppy, or a sick or old dog, or a dog which has problems with it's pancreas. Apart from that, unless a dog has an allergy to eggs, there should be no problem.
- The second problem is that egg whites contain a substance called AVIDIN, which binds with the vitamin biotin [a member of the B complex], making it unavailable for your dog. The only situation where this has been a problem was when an experimental diet, totally deficient in biotin was fed together with lots of raw egg whites for several weeks.

The only likely possibility I know of where lots of egg whites could precipitate a biotin deficiency, would be where a dog was fed a poor quality dried dog food. If that dry food was low in biotin, as they often are, the dog may suffer a biotin deficiency.

Another reason for confidence is that egg yolks contain plenty of biotin, so that feeding whole eggs is very safe. For example, egg flips... made from whole eggs and milk have been a favourite invalid food for generations causing health, not a biotin deficiency.

● We know a fox. He loves RAW eggs. Probably gets one nearly every day... and guess what ...... no biotin deficiency.

So forget it.... the whole idea of RAW eggs being dangerous as part of a balanced diet is absurd.

If you are having a problem with the whites, you can cook them. That eliminates both problems. However, do not cook the yolks, continue to feed them raw.

In other words, unless you know your dog cannot tolerate egg whites, go ahead and feed whole raw eggs as PART of your adult healthy dog's natural balanced diet.

How do You Use Eggs to Feed Dogs ?

The simplest way to think of eggs is as a BRILLIANT PRO-TEIN supplement, and when you use it... you get the added bonus of all those other nutrients, such as vitamin A, the B vitamins, and most particularly the calcium and the essential fatty acids, the iron and the zinc and the enzymes and other longevity factors always present in whole raw foods. Note that because it is a whole unprocessed food it gives your dog more nutrients than we are aware of. This is as opposed to processed "scientifically balanced" foods. The so called "complete" dog foods. All you get with these is problems. Anyway, back to using eggs.

● Let me repeat that whenever you want to add protein to a dish for your dog.. one of the best things you can add is an egg. One of the great things about eggs is that they are liquid. This makes them so easy to combine with other foods.

In our household, they are commonly added to a vegetable dish to boost the protein content, or to milk. Our dogs love them ! Often we whisk in some brewer's yeast. Alternatively, we just give them the whole egg.

Think of Protein - Think of Eggs

It is their ability to provide high quality protein at a cheap price which makes eggs such a wonderful food. There are times in a dog's life when exta protein is absolutely essential. For example, eggs are brilliant food for nursing mothers, growing puppies, pregnant mums and for older dogs where you wish to provide good quality protein in small amounts.

Egg yolks are an essential food for a dog with skin problems. They contain sulphur containing amino acids, biotin, vitamin A, essential fatty acids and zinc.

- The bottom line is, when you need to supply high quality protein that is rich in many other nutrients... at a cheap price, think of eggs.

- 15 -

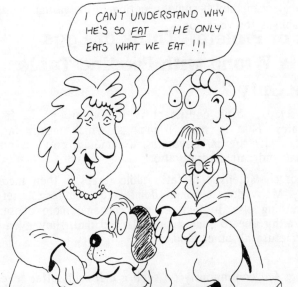

Table Scraps as Dog Food

Most vets advise against feeding table scraps to dogs. They also add that if table scraps are fed, they should comprise no more than twenty five percent of the dog's total food intake. This is based on the assumption that the bulk of the diet is commercial dog food.

- If you do feed mostly commercial dog food, then your
  vet's advice is sound. Those artificial commercial dog food
  diets are very fragile. That is, very easily unbalanced. The
  more table scraps that are added to them, the more
  unbalanced they become, resulting in increasing health
  problems for your dog.

What is Wrong with Feeding Table Scraps Only ?

Table scraps mostly consist of two food groups ..... fat and
carbohydrates. That is, meat trimmings, which means fat, and
vegetables, which are carbohydrates. Commonly, gravy is present,
which is fat and carbohydrate also.

A major characteristic of fatty table scraps is their incredible
palatability. Many dogs become addicted to such food..... refusing
to eat anything else. In fact, as they become more obese, and
more unhealthy due to such an unbalanced diet, they even more
stubbornly refuse all other food.

- Dogs fed continuously on such a diet will suffer severe
  malnutrition in the form of a deficiency of protein,
     minerals, often the essential fatty acids, and vitamins.

Such a diet would rapidly cause stunting, growth and bone
problems in a growing pup, and in an adult dog will cause
obesity to start with, but has the potential to produce just about
every conceivable health problem a dog could possibly develop.
This includes cancer and other degenerative diseases, including
diseases of the pancreas, particularly Pancreatitis. Other organs
that will suffer include the liver, the heart and possibly the kidneys.

I am talking here about a situation where people feed the fat
trimmings to their dog to total excess. A few are OK with other
foods. Please also note at this point that if your hard working
dog is fed lots of fat to give it extra energy, do feed extra vitamin E.

Balancing Table Scraps

Your vet is very happy for you to feed table scraps to your dog so long as you know how to balance them using readily available healthy foods.

- Just remember, you cannot balance table scraps by using commercially produced dog food, because as I have said, it is an artificial food, so it's balance is delicate and easily upset.

If we go back thirty or forty years, most dogs were fed on the family's left overs together with bones and scraps of meat from the butcher. If you listen to people who can remember back that far, they will tell you how dogs fed that way did very well. Those dogs had no need of vets. Mind you, that was fortunate, because vets were hard to find in those days.

The good news is, our dogs have not changed. It's only been a few decades. We can still go back to that style of feeding, but we can now do it with much more nutritional knowledge.

Of course in some instances the scraps might have changed. It is likely that today's scraps will contain a high proportion of un-wholesome fast junk food.

- The best way to approach our table scraps or left overs, is to make a quick assessment of what they mainly consist of, and see what else we need to feed our dog in order to give it a balanced diet, keeping in mind that balance does not have to be, and indeed should not be achieved at every meal.

Let us return to that worst scenario. The feeding of dogs on table scraps consisting mostly of fatty trimmings, gravy and car-bohydrate rich vegetables.

By feeding your dog such food, - cooked - mostly what you have supplied is energy. Your dog misses out on all the nutrients only available from raw food such as enzymes and anti-oxidants etc.. It also lacks adequate protein, possibly essential fatty acids, and there will not be enough minerals and vitamins.

Raw Meaty Bones to the Rescue !

The bulk of those deficiencies can be remedied with one cheap easily available product. The raw meaty bone. Bones are the perfect mineral source for your dog. Raw meaty bones fill in most of the other gaps as well ! That is, they supply proteins, the essential fatty acids, many of the nutrients only available from raw foods, and some of the fat soluble vitamins. Add some green leafy vegetables, organ meats, brewer's yeast, eggs etc. and hey presto, the diet is balanced. It really is that simple.

Another way, apart from raw bones, to get calcium and other minerals into your dog is to feed dairy foods, and legumes. However, I strongly advise you not to rely on these products to supply your dog's mineral requirements. Stick to the raw meaty bone, they are cheaper, and do a far better job.

You do not have to feed the bones and the scraps at the same sitting. In fact I would strongly advise against the practice. Most table scraps will be more available at night after the main meal of the day. Feed them then. Throw in some brewers yeast [the B vitamins] and a kelp tablet [iodine], and you are done.

Give your dog it's meaty bones in the morning. That should keep it occupied all day.

You can vary all this of course. Suppose the bones your dog had one morning were not very meaty, and the only scraps that night was a bit of left over rice. In that case, you might add some baked beans or throw in a couple of eggs and perhaps some pulverised vegetable scraps and a small amount of vegetable oil, etc..

If using table scraps consisting mostly of grain products and vegetable left overs, and the only bones being used are beef or lamb, you may need to add one of the vegetable oils to the scraps to make sure there are sufficient essential fatty acids present.

Do Not Feed too Much Cooked Food

When including table scraps as part of your dog's diet, it is important to guard against feeding mostly cooked food. Naturally the bones you feed will be raw, but do ensure that the rest of the diet consists of at the very least, fifty percent raw foods.

One way to do this is to use the vegetable peelings. They actually contain more food value than the inside bits. Wash them well to remove any toxic chemicals before peeling them, and then put them through the juicer or the blender etc., to reduce them to pulp before feeding them to your dog.

If you wish to feed your dog a totally natural diet, feeding cooked table scraps is out. Feed the raw ones only. I assume they will be mostly vegetable matter. If that is the case, see the section on feeding vegetables to your dog. Apart from that, the advice is no different. Base the diet on raw meaty bones and add eggs, oils, kelp and brewer's yeast etc..

Conclusion

Basically, no matter what the scraps are, so long as they are supplemented with plenty of RAW MEATY BONES..... you cannot go too far wrong. Just keep in mind that dogs eat everything, and that the best way to ensure balance is to feed a wide variety of other foods, particularly raw foods.

You can Help our Planet

Also keep in mind, that when you use your table scraps, vegetable peelings etc. to feed the dog, rather than throwing them out with the garbage, you are doing something to save money and conserve energy. By feeding table scraps to the dog we are recycling otherwise useless food.

If we multiply the savings made by one household feeding left overs to their dog[s], by all the dog owning families potentially able to do this, we can see the possibility of making an incredible saving of the energy reserves of our over-populated, under-resourced planet.

This chapter should be read in conjunction with chapter 18 if you are feeding an adult dog, chapter 17 if feeding a puppy, or chapter 22 if feeding an older dog.

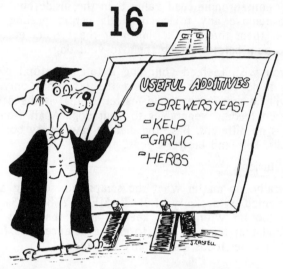

16

Useful Additives

If you are feeding mostly raw meaty bones to your dog and not much else as so many people do, then it is essential that you supply two supplements on a regular basis. One of these is brewers yeast and the other is kelp.

BREWER'S YEAST

• The overriding reason this is added to your dog's diet is as a source of the B complex group of vitamins.

What is brewer's yeast ? For a start, and this is important, it is not baker's yeast. Baker's yeast is living yeast. The one you use to make bread rise. Baker's yeast will deprive your dog of B vitamins, as opposed to brewer's yeast which supplies them. Nor is it the living yeast used to make home brew beer.

Brewer's yeast is composed of the dead bodies of yeast organisms. It is a pasteurised residue of commercial brewed beer. It can also be grown especially for use as a food.

- It is one of the richest, most concentrated sources of nutrients known.
- By supplying your dog with brewer's yeast on a regular basis, you go a long way towards providing him or her with many of the nutrients dogs in the wild obtain by eating faeces, plus some other benefits besides.

There is a very similar product called Torula yeast, the major difference being that Torula Yeast is much lower in sodium, and is therefore useful in cases where a low sodium intake is required such as in heart or kidney disease. Another difference is that Torula yeast has double the fibre and calcium content of brewer's yeast.

The Nutrients in Brewer's Yeast

Brewers yeast is high in both protein and carbohydrates, containing about 40 % of each. It is very low in fats.

- It is one of the richest sources of the B complex group of vitamins, being particularly rich in vitamin B1 or Thiamin. It has reasonable levels of B2 or Riboflavin, high levels of B3 or Nicotinic acid, excellent levels of B5 or Calcium Pantothenate, with Pyridoxine or B6, Biotin, Folic acid, P.A.B.A. and Pangamic acid all present at reasonable levels.
- The minerals it contains include in order of abundance, potassium, phosphorus, magnesium, calcium, sodium and iron. The iron levels in brewer's yeast are two to three times those found in beef. Note that it contains eight times more phosphorus than calcium.
- Brewer's yeast is a rich source of both DNA and RNA... which is why there is such a high phosphorus content.
- Brewer's yeast contains a CHROMIUM compound called glucose tolerance factor or GTF. This compound is vital in preventing adult onset diabetes. It does this by keeping your dog's blood sugar levels on an even keel. This is particularly important in dogs receiving the highly

diabetogenic diets of today... that is the commercial processed foods with their high levels of starch, their added simple soluble sugars, and the very common practice of feeding sugar-laden tit-bits such as cakes and biscuits and chocolates and ice cream to our dogs.

Adding brewer's yeast to the diet of diabetic dogs will help reduce their need for insulin. Other chromium rich foods include chicken, shell fish, meat, mushrooms, whole grain, beer, and corn oil.

- Brewer's yeast also contains SELENIUM. As recently as twenty years ago, we had no idea of the importance of this mineral to the general health of all animals. We knew it was important to protect calves and lambs against white muscle disease, but that was about it.

Today we realise it's vital importance in protecting dogs against cancer, heart disease, and stroke. Like it's anti-oxidant partners, the vitamins A, C and E, selenium is a powerful weapon in slowing down the ageing processes in your dog. It helps your dog's tissues retain their youthful elasticity, and helps in the production of antibodies. Low selenium in your dog's diet means a poorly functioning immune system.

Selenium is essential for optimal sexual functioning in male dogs. It is important in arthritis treatment and in preventing cataracts.

Selenium is also found in celery, onions, radishes, broccoli, cucumbers, garlic, eggs, mushroom, seafood, liver, meat, kidneys, and whole grains. Most natural selenium is destroyed by cooking and modern processing.

KELP

This is the name given to many different varieties of large seaweeds. It is a valuable source of a number of minerals, but most particularly IODINE. It contains 15 % sodium, 13 % potassium, 3 % calcium, with trace amounts of IODINE, manganese, magnesium, copper, phosphorus, zinc, cobalt, chromium and molybdenum.

How Much Kelp ?

A kelp tablet daily for your average 20 kg dog will ensure it gets adequate iodine for the functioning of the thyroid gland. This is essential for growing puppies, reproducing animals and for all other dogs. A healthy, well nourished [with iodine] thyroid ensures your dog's metabolism ticks over at the right speed.

Other good sources of iodine are seafoods and dairy foods. The dairy foods are usually good sources because of the iodine based disinfectants used in their production. Vegetables will be rich in iodine to the extent that the soil they are grown in contains iodine. In Australia, iodine can be lacking in many soils.

- Over-zealous administration of iodine can be toxic to your dog. It causes the thyroid to shut down production of thyroid hormone and your dog's whole metabolism slows down.

- I suspect bones are also a good source of iodine because I have raised many dogs on raw meaty bones with very little of anything else, and there have been no problems with those dogs so far as their thyroid function was concerned.

GARLIC

This is probably one of the most useful herbs you can feed to your dog. You can feed a clove or two or more daily depending on the size of your dog and how close you and the dog are.. in terms of the way your dog will smell. I guess it will be OK if you are eating plenty as well.

There is no doubt that garlic eating does confer some health advantages. If your dog eats sufficient garlic often enough it will help stabilise blood pressure and give a good solid boost to the immune system, keeping at bay infections of various sorts particularly upper respiratory tract infections. Much of it's success is due to various compounds of sulphur.

Garlic has often been used to good effect with dogs that have problems with fleas. Fleas tend to inhabit the bodies of unhealthy dogs. I do not know whether it was because the garlic made the dog healthier and therefore less attractive to fleas, or whether it just acted as a flea repellant. In any case, many clients have reported a great drop in flea problems once they started to feed garlic to their dogs.

Perhaps the most acceptable way to feed garlic to your dog is as the fermented and aged "Kyolic" garlic. This has the advantage of being unlikely to cause stomach upsets when fed in large amounts compared to raw garlic fed straight from the garden.

- Be wary of other forms of processed garlic. They may no longer have the active ingredients present.

OTHER HERBS

There are many other herbs which you could feed to your dog with great advantage. It would appear that a major function of many herbs is to supply much needed anti-oxidants to the person or animal consuming them. They certainly can be very useful in treating disease processes. However, that information would fill another book, so rather than do such an important topic an injustice, I shall not discuss them further.

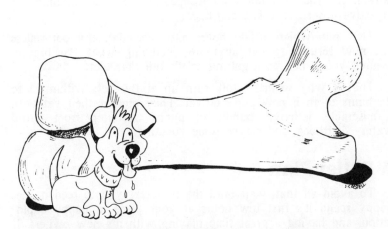

17

Feeding Your New Puppy

AT LAST I HAVE MY NEW PUPPY !

Most folk, as soon as they get their new puppy home want to feed it straight away. Usually that is not a great idea. My advice is, if you must feed the pup, do do not let it eat a lot. If it is allowed to eat as much as it wants to, which a lot of new owners just love to see, it drastically overeats. It eats as if it had never been fed before. It overeats because it is used to competing with a heap of hungry puppies for food.

That new puppy has no idea it has been removed from it's mum, it's brothers and sisters, from the humans it was used to, and from the surroundings, which it loved and called home.

Sometime in the next 24 hours all this will dawn on your new puppy. The realisation of being lost and lonely and miserable. Meanwhile, with all that food in it's little tummy, particularly if it's food it's not used to, you will almost certainly see digestive upsets, colic and diarrhoea.

That pup which a few hours ago seemed like a bottomless pit, now refuses to eat anything, including what the breeder assured you it had been getting as it's full time diet.

That is why so many folk turn up at the vets within 12 to 24 hours of their new pup's arrival. They present their vet with a miserable, lethargic bundle of puppy suffering from putrid watery diarrhoea, and maybe some vomiting.

A Better Plan

To avoid all that, wait until the pup asks you to feed it. Let puppy spend it's first few hours at your place in happy exploration, and having a great time playing with it's new owners. If it wants to drink water... no problem.. let it find the bowl you have casually placed on the floor.

This ensures that pup gets to know you and it's new home on a casual relaxed basis. Exploring and playing is tiring for a pup. There is a very good chance your new pup will sleep through the first night with no disturbance. You can help that along with a drink of milk, egg and honey. [See recipe in chapter 13]

The next morning, that hungry little pup will be happy to accept the food you offer.

The first food we offer all new pups are chicken wings, or at least some sort of boney off cuts. I cannot think of one occasion when a hungry new puppy was not prepared to eat a chicken wing or similar, and always with great enthusiasm.

However, as I have said, do not let it gorge itself. You may offer another in a few hours, but still leave it hungry. This way it will quickly settle into its new home with very few tummy or psychological upsets.

The important point is not to give it too much. If you know the sort of food it had been eating before coming to your place, that will be OK for the moment.

In a few hours, offer some more of the same, but still leave it hungry. This way it will quickly settle into it's new home with very few tummy or psychological upsets. If you wish to change puppy's diet, you may do so after puppy has settled in.

That Brings us to a Most Important Question

Apart from what the breeder may or may not have told you to feed that puppy, just what sort of food do puppies eat ?

Do you give it cat food ? That sounds all right. Should you feed it mince ? A lot of folk do. What about milk, porridge, eggs? Can it eat bones ? How about some rice, left over veggies and a bit of gravy, or that bit of chicken from last night's tea ? Perhaps some breakfast cereal ? What about steak or kangaroo meat from the pet shop ? Will this bit of custard do any harm ? Then there is ice cream, and chocolates, and bread, and butter, and vegemite ? What about fruit and yoghurt and cream ? What about commercially produced "scientifically balanced", needs-nothing-else-added, straight-from-a-tin-or-packet puppy food ? That might be easiest.

The truth is, you can feed your puppy all or some of the above or something entirely different. The choices are in fact, almost endless for your opportunist, carnivorous, omnivorous, sca-venging puppy.

In other words, your puppy can and will eat just about any-thing, but what is the absolute best ?

● This is the most important choice you will make for your new puppy.

Yes, I know you will keep it away from other dogs until it is fully vaccinated for Distemper, Hepatitis and Parvovirus. You will worm it regularly, and take great care not to run over it or tread on it. You will groom it and teach it good manners. You will make sure it does not get heartworm. However, the big question is, will you feed it properly ? Do you know how to feed it properly ?

● The way you feed your new puppy will determine it's health for the rest of it's life. It is that important.

Most new puppy owners seem to know this as if by instinct.

That is why they plague their vet with questions like.......

"What is the best food to feed my puppy ?

What is the best brand of puppy food ?

How often should my puppy be fed ?

How much should my puppy be fed ?

What sort of meat should I feed my puppy ?

Should you feed puppies bones ?

If so what sort ?

What about calcium?

What sort and how much?

What about food scraps ?

Is cat food OK?

My puppy is a Chihuahua, does it have special needs?

My puppy is a Great Dane, I suppose it needs lots of extra calcium?".

The questions are never ending. People with new puppies do not only ask vets of course. They seek and are given advice from every quarter.

- It is not surprising that so many people are unsure about feeding dogs, particularly puppies. They receive a mass of confusing and often conflicting hints coming at them from all directions. From breeders, pet shop owners, adverts on television, vets, books, butchers, newspaper articles and so on.

Who Should They Believe ?

The answer to that is very simple. To get the answers you need, you have to ask the dog itself. The way to do that is to observe three things. What happens in nature, what happens in families and kennels all over the world as different puppy feeding regimes are tried, and the results of modern research into canine nutrition.

By understanding what puppies eat in the wild, you will have valuable clues as to what we should be feeding our domestic pup of today. You will find out exactly what the digestive system of a pup is programmed to eat by centuries of evolution.

Combine that approach with an examination of the results of modern research together with feeding trials... carried out daily all over the world, in the homes of new puppy owners, and you will get first hand practical advice on what works well today, and what doesn't.

Your Puppy has the Insides of a Wolf

We cannot be absolutely certain about the origins of the domestic dog. One thing is for sure. Your little puppy came originally from wild dogs, and there is a lot of evidence to suggest that wild dog may have been the wolf.

Although we humans have changed the appearance and the nature of the dog in all sorts of ways by domestication, we have not changed it's basic internal workings. In other words, today's domestic dog has essentially the same digestive system and over all physiology as it's ancestor the wolf.

That is why it is valid to study what wolves and other wild dogs eat, to help develop a healthy puppy diet today.

- This approach is used by all modern zoos and by hospitals which use animals in their fight against human disease. As much as is possible, all the animals in these places are fed their natural diet, and this includes the dogs. No processed food here. Zoologists know that natural foods produces the greatest health with the least problems.

Wolf Cubs Growing Up.

By looking at young wolves growing up, we are actually observing our young puppy's ancestors. If we couple that with our modern scientific discoveries about diet, health and ageing, we should be able to produce a realistic, health promoting, puppy diet.

Wolf cubs grow up hungry, they grow slowly and they eat a lot of bones. They spend their day in play, in sleeping, in scavenging, and eating. Eating little bits all the time, and bigger meals as food becomes available. They are not fed on any sort of regular basis. Sometimes they go for a couple of days without much food.

All their food is raw. Nothing is cooked. That single fact is vitally important. Wild dogs eat totally raw food all the time. Their whole digestive system, their whole physiology demands raw food.

- Your puppy is no different. For your puppy's health sake, most of it's food should be raw.

Wild puppies eat or try to eat just about everything they come across. This includes soil, the stomach contents of their parent's prey, mostly chewed up and fermenting grass; raw meat, raw bones, raw offal such as heart, kidneys, brains, eyes etc; raw vegetables, raw fruit, raw grass, raw berries, raw insects, raw bark, raw roots, raw faeces etc.. You name it and they eat it or try to eat it. All raw, nothing cooked.

Young wolf cubs do not seriously hunt. They play. When they have finished playing they stop and rest. No long boring walks on a lead for wolf cubs......

In the wolf family, eating is based strictly on an individual's position in the pecking order, or order of dominance. When times are tough, a wolf who is low on the pecking order goes hungry. This is important when it comes to understanding how to feed domestic puppies.

Weaned wolf puppies, puppies abandoned by mum, are left to fend for themselves. They are at the bottom of the pecking order. This means they are the last ones to eat. No preferential treatment like our modern pups.

- Those half starved puppies, fighting amongst themselves do not get to eat a lot. Mostly, it is whatever the adults leave. The result is that what they do manage to eat, the central theme of their diet is raw meaty bones, and not much else.

The "not much else" is important however. It includes

material such as bits and pieces of internal organs, bits of intestines with their finely crushed grass and other vegetation-type-contents, some faeces, and whatever else they can find that seems remotely edible.

The pup's hunger is important. Firstly, it drives those wild puppies to supplement and balance their diet by scavenging and hunting. They learn to eat a wide array of food types. Whatever they find in the way of fruit, insects, roots, edible fungi, soil, berries, grass, etc. they eat. The second thing it ensures, is that they never grow at their maximum pace.

- From studying the eating habits of wolf cubs which are seen to be perpetually hungry, subsisting on raw food consisting mostly of bones and being forced to scavenge a wide variety of foods, we get four vital clues about successful puppy raising.

Four Vital Clues

- Number one... The bulk of a puppy's diet should consist of raw meaty bones.
- Number two... all or most of the rest of their food should also be raw.
- Number three... Puppies should always be kept hungry. They should never be grown at their maximum growth rate. They should be kept slim, lean and hard. Guard against roly poly, fat, young puppies.
- Number four... puppies should learn to eat everything.

Let us Look at some Modern Feeding Experiments

Ironically, it is usually those people who are most determined to do the absolute best job of feeding their puppy, that make the most mistakes and produce the poorest results.

- Doting owners, using "the very best food" and plenty of
  it together with lots of calcium supplements, produce
  rapidly growing puppies .. and ... exactly what they did
  not want, a puppy with problems. However, others,
  people who don't try too hard, but follow their nose,
  often end up doing an excellent job. Let us see why that
  is.

I want you to consider two typical puppy raising scenarios.
We vets get to see such dramas played out on an almost daily
basis. I am going to describe to you the raising of two pups.
Both were Rottweilers, they were from the same litter, they
were both females, and both appeared to be in perfect health
when they went to their new home.

One of the pups was bought by a young truck driver. He
was married with a couple of kids. It was a spur of the moment
decision. He thought the dog would be great to guard his truck.
He left the job of rearing it to the lady of the house.

The other one was delivered to the home of a wealthy young
business couple. They were planning to have it as a show dog,
and possibly as some sort of status symbol.

Raising the Truckie's Rottie - or
The Puppy that Brings Itself Up.....

Harried young mother, three screaming kids, a hardworking,
never-at-home husband, and a brand new puppy. Dad hopes it
will guard his truck.. eventually. He is wrong of course. it will
end up belonging to mum and the kids.

You see, mother gets the job of rearing it, and dogs tend to
love and give their loyalty to the one who feeds and looks after,
and with kindness, disciplines them.

It is said that if you want anything done, give it to a busy
person. That is what happened in this case. Along with shopping, feeding the kids, doing the housework, washing, ironing,
cooking, cleaning etc. etc., all on a fairly limited budget, this
young lady was also expected to raise the puppy.

A busy mum has not got a lot of time for a young pup.

However, using her common sense, and trusting in luck, she does the best she can.

Let's examine what that typical young mother with limited resources feeds a young seven week old puppy that is suddenly thrust upon her.....

- Those food scraps the kids didn't eat will do. Get some bones from the butcher. That'll keep it busy and out from under mum's feet. Drop it the unwanted food scraps while preparing the human's food.

- Forget about the dog food, it's expensive, besides, that canned stuff stinks and it tends to give puppy the trots ! Bones are cheap, and the scraps cost nothing.

- Puppy occasionally raids the garbage can, the kitchen tidy, eats the cat droppings in the sand pit and the kitty litter, and anything else it can find which seems remotely like food.

A neglected pup ? Perhaps, perhaps not. Strangely enough, it seems to be growing up fine, with no problems ! However, before we pass final judgement, consider the following.

Puppy that Gets the Best of Everything

We are now in the home of that wealthy young business couple. They have just taken delivery of their brand new puppy.

This moment has been planned for some time. They have been to dog shows and breeders too numerous to mention. Finally bought this pup before it was even conceived! Waiting, waiting, waiting... throughout the pregnancy, through the young puppy sucking on mother stage, and finally, at long last the day arrives. At long last they have their beautiful new Rottie puppy.

- Every thing is ready. They have a brand spanking new kennel, they have puppy food by the truck load, freezers full of expensive steak, they have vitamin supplements, they have mineral supplemenmts, especially calcium, and they have the phone number of absolutely every vet in town......... just in case.

Every waking moment is devoted to that pup. Every breath puppy draws is analysed and every action observed. Every motion that puppy passes is examined for colour, consistency, smell, size, weight, texture. All abnormalities are noted, and the vet rung or visited at great expense to enquire the significance of these happenings

This puppy is going to be the best in town. It is going to grow bigger and faster, and have stronger bones than any other puppy ever. Three square meals a day. May be four. Look at this pup grow. It is big and fat and roly and shiny and beeootiful. Calcium supplements are poured into this pup. It's bones are going to be perfect. Only the best is good enough for this puppy. No expense is spared.

Every care is taken to ensure that nothing untoward happens to this puppy. It is never allowed to eat soil, or the droppings of other animals. Such things contain germs and worms, and could well do it harm. At least that is the reason the owners give if asked.

● Also, and this is most important, this puppy is not
   allowed to chew bones. It's owners believe they are
   positively dangerous.

Every piece of food it is given is cut up into small tempting morsels which ensures puppy eats as much as possible. To further enhance this eating frenzy, all food is beautifuly cooked. This means more of it is eaten, because it tastes better than raw food, and also, it ensures all possible parasites and germs are totally destroyed.

Puppy is not allowed any scraps of any description, because it is on a strict growth diet of carefully selected lean meats, vitamin and mineral supplements, and top quality dog foods. No chances will be taken with this pup.

Exercise ? Is this puppy exercised ! This puppy will be no weakling. It is going to be developed into a champion right from the start. Every morning and afternoon, out on the lead, off we go for a good long healthy walk, to make sure that lungs and heart and muscle and bones and nerves are all developed to the peak of perfection.

- The owners strongly believe that this puppy will be perfectly healthy and win all the shows. But will she ?

Fortunately this pups owners are very wealthy. They need to be. For some unexplained reason, even though it was bought from a stud where it's parents had been certified as free from all hereditary bone diseases, including hip dysplasia, before it reached the age of four months of age, this puppy was having difficulty walking.

Several vets are consulted. In the end, a specialist is visited. Practically every major joint in the body is affected. They are told by the specialist that this is the worst case he has ever seen.

- By the time that pup is nine months old, more than two thousand dollars have been spent on her with vets and specialist attention.
- Meanwhile the only money spent at the vets on the other pup is for worming and vaccination. Just a normal, happy, healthy pup.

The Winner

It may seem strange, but out of the two pups I have just described, the pup which had all the fuss made over it, the one that ate all the expensive food and calcium supplements, the one that had all that care taken, all that money spent on it including all that top class veterinary attention, by the time it reaches adult hood does not turn out to be the healthiest of the two. Far from it.

- In fact, at age three, that dog had to be put down because of crippling arthritis.

The dog which is brought up amidst the hurly burly life of a young family, the dog which practically brings itself up, living on a diet of bones, food scraps, and whatever else it can find, and playing with the kids in the backyard, will in most cases grow to adulthood with very few problems.

Why is This ?

Surely the more care we take of our young puppy, the healthier he will be ? That is common sense - yes ? True enough, if the care you take is the right sort of care.

- However, it is possible to literally kill or maim your young puppy with kindness.

We vets see the disasterous results of over-zealous, trying-too-hard-to-do-the-right- thing type puppy rearing all the time.

- ALL the common bone problems seen in young pups including hip dysplasia are the result of incorrect feeding and exercise of the type the pampered over fed puppy received.
- This is true of obesity, skin problems, dental problems, and a host of other problems that occur as the life of the dog progresses. It also includes the old age diseases. Such things as diabetes, heart disease, arthritis, cancer and so on.

I want to pause for a moment, and examine what that harried young mother did for that puppy which was soooooo right ...

The Puppy Raising Secrets of a Young Mother

Why is it that a young mother, with no training, no help from anyone, quite a lot of distractions and very little money for expensive foods or supplements, managed to successfully rear a young pup of one of the larger breeds ? Breeds which are notorious for developing bone problems if not raised carefully.

How did this young mother do so well, seemingly without really trying ?

- That young mother actually duplicated many of the conditions under which her puppy's ancestors, wolves,

were raised, for countless generations. A process that has
continued for literally millions of years, long before man
came on the scene, and tried, with the help of science
and commercial dog food, to do better.

Lack of time and money helped. It ensured that pup was fed
lots of bones. When mum gave that pup a meaty bone to eat,
she knew it would not bother her for a couple of hours at least.

THAT IS THE FIRST AND MOST IMPORTANT SECRET
FOR SUCCESS IN PUPPY REARING. BONES. That puppy ate
a lot of bones, just like it's ancestors, the wolf cubs.

- What she did not realise, was the enormous benefits,
  nutritional, physical, dental and psychological she was
  giving to that pup when she fed it bones.

Not that it mattered whether she realised or not. She had
done it, and that was the main thing. In fact, that habit of toss-
ing bones to her puppy on a regular basis, that is, practically
every day, is the first and most important secret for success in
puppy rearing. Bones.

- Because that puppy ate a lot of raw meaty bones, just
  like it's ancestors, the wolf cubs, this was a guarantee,
  the closest you can get to a guarantee when rearing
  pups, that this one would be healthy.

Lack of time and money also helped ensure that puppy was
fed sparingly, just like the wolf cubs. Sure it was fed adequately, but it was not over fed on a regular basis. This is the:-

SECOND SECRET OF SUCCESSFUL PUPPY REARING..

The puppy never grew at it's maximum growth rate. It was
never one of those roly poly fat puppies.

- It is a general scientific principle that any plant or animal
  grown at it's maximum growth rate is much more prone
  to disease, is short lived and in general is much less
  healthy than animals or plants which are held back. Not
  stunted, just held back slightly.

The held back creatures still grow as big, it just takes a bit
longer.

This brings us to the:-

THIRD SECRET OF SUCCESSFUL PUPPY REARING used by that young mother. Because puppy was hungry much of the time, and because mum did not have a lot of time for it, that pup did lots of scavenging. It ate all manner of things. These included grass, cat droppings, insects, it's own droppings, scraps from the table, bones it had previously buried, and of course soil.

In other words, the third secret of successful puppy rearing used by that young mother was that she gave the puppy plenty of opportunity to eat a wide variety of foods. Just like it's ancestors the wolves.

- The greater the range of foods that pups become
  acustomed to and learn to eat, the greater the chance
  they will get all the nutrients they need for healthy
  growth and development. In later life, pups fed this way
  continue to accept a wide range of foods and thereby
  maintain their health.

THE FOURTH SUCCESS SECRET used by this young mother was to feed the pup a lot of raw food. Like the wolf cub, that puppy's body is designed to do best on raw food. Science has discovered a whole host of nutrients in raw food which are essential to health and longevity.

- These nutrients are destroyed during cooking. They
  include vitamins, enzymes and many other compounds
  with life-extending and health-promoting properties under
  the general name of anti-oxidants. While the vitamins can
  be replaced with supplements, most of the others are only
  found in raw food.

If we can feed raw foods to pups without endangering human health [see Chapter 9] and without endangering our dogs' health, then we should do so. The results will not always be apparent immediately, [they often are], but over a period of years, the difference in the health of dogs raised on raw foods compared to those raised on cooked foods is staggering.

- Of course there are foods such as grains which must be
  fed cooked, but in general, raw food is what your puppy
  requires.

THE FIFTH SECRET OF SUCCESS used to rear that puppy occurred because it lived with a young growing family. That puppy was fed food suitable for growth. That is, high energy food, high protein food, and food rich in vitamins and minerals.

Basically, if those young kids were on a healthy type of growth diet, then so was the dog as it ate the scraps and the left overs from their table.

- The sort of food I am talking about includes such things as eggs, oatmeal porridge, yoghurt, vegetables, meat scraps, cheese, whole meal bread etc..

THE SIXTH SECRET OF SUCCESS in raising this young puppy, relates to the fact that the family was struggling, and not awfully rich. This puppy was fed on butcher's bones and left overs. The owners could not afford and possibly did not even know about calcium supplements. They certainly would not buy loads of expensive high class meat for the pup. They did not use dog food.

In other words, the sixth success secret used by that young mother was not to use a combination of calcium supplements, commercial dog foods and loads of expensive steak as the basis of that puppy's diet.

- More puppies in the last 10 to 20 years, have been ruined by a diet of commercial dog food, expensive steak and calcium than perhaps any other method.

THE SEVENTH SUCCESS SECRET was the way this young puppy received it's exercise. Mother did not have time to take puppy for long interminable walks twice daily. Instead, puppy romped with it's "brothers and sisters", the kids, in the back yard. It simply played. When it had had enough, it stopped. Just like the wolf cubs.

- One of the major causes of bone problems in adult dogs is the sort of exercise they receive when young. The problems I refer to include hip dysplasia, elbow displasia, shoulder dysplasia etc..

Those long boring walks result in a tired and bored puppy which can hardly drag itself along. Bones previously held strongly by taut strong muscles, no longer have this protection. They now grind heavily against each other ... this process helping to remould their soft ends... Part of the formula for bone problems !

THE EIGHTH SECRET of successful puppy rearing relates to this young mother's inability and unwillingness to keep puppy inside. That young puppy had access to sunlight, fresh air, grass, plants, insects, soil and plenty of fresh water.

THE NINTH SUCCESS SECRET used by that young mother was not trying to give her puppy everything it needed in a nutritional sense, in each and every meal. She raised it the common sense way, the way she raised her kids. She achieved balance for that puppy by feeding a wide variety of foods at many different meals.

She may not have known it, but it is actually much more beneficial to a pup if individual meals concentrate on a limited range of foods. The major reason for this is to prevent interaction by different nutrients which tend to become unavailable or indigestible, particularly when they are also cooked.

- The attempt to make each meal balanced and complete is a major problem inherent in all modern processed foods.

THE TENTH SECRET OF SUCCESS used by this young mother was to do it with lots of love thrown in. That love, that interest, ensures two vital things. Firstly, the psychological effect of being loved and wanted, helps build a strong immune system in the pup. Secondly, it ensures that the puppy is "looked at" on a regular daily basis.

- LOOKING at growing pups is vitally important. It helps to decide how much food should be fed. For example .... "No more food for you today my young puppy... you are getting too fat !"... or... "Oops, did I forget to feed you last night, here, have another chicken wing !"
- By studying this mum's methods in the light of rearing wolf cubs in the wild, we find that we have discovered the.....

Ten Secrets of Successful Puppy Rearing

FIRST SECRET.. Heaps of raw meaty bones as the basis and major component of the diet..... about 60 % of total food intake.

- SECOND SECRET.. Grow those pups slowly, keeping them lean and slightly hungry.
- THIRD SECRET.. Feed those pups a wide variety of foods.
- FOURTH SECRET.. Feed those pups mostly raw foods.
- FIFTH SECRET.. Feed foods suitable for growth, that is, high in good quality protein, fats, vitamins and minerals.
- SIXTH SECRET.. Do not base the diet of those puppies on raw steak, commercial dog food and calcium supplements.
- SEVENTH SECRET.. The only exercise allowed is play.
- EIGHTH SECRET.. Pups must spend most of their day outside in the fresh air on clean earth and grass in the sun, with ample fresh water available.
- NINTH SECRET.. The diet is to be balanced over time, not by providing balance in every meal.
- The TENTH SECRET.. is a puppy raised with love, resulting in a strong immune system, and a puppy that is "watched", and fed according to it's weight, condition and general health.

The Importance of Bones .. or Getting Down to First Principles !

- What I want to stress is the absolute importance of raw meaty bones to your growing puppy. It is essential to build your puppy's diet around raw meaty bones. With them your pup will grow easily and well and will have no problems. Without them, we vets see a continual parade of horrors in terms of puppy health.

If you decide to go the meat [and no bones] and supplement route.... you will almost certainly fail, and if you decide on going the all commercial dog food way... well, the pup will go OK .... PROBABLY... for a while, but in the long term, if that is all you feed.. you will produce an adult dog with a multitude of problems.

Raw Meaty Bones Supply Most of a Puppy's Nutritional Needs

Your puppy needs food that will support it's proper growth. It is most important that you understand the importance of bones in this regard. It's requirements include adequate protein, fat, energy, vitamins and minerals. Raw meaty bones do in fact supply most of those requirements.

The very best raw meaty bones in our experience are chicken wings, or chicken necks. They supply top quality protein, top quality fat, the fat soluble vitamins, some of the B vitamins, plenty of energy, and all the minerals your pup requires, and this may include iodine.

The fat in raw chicken has an excellent balance of essential fatty acids plus the fat soluble vitamins your puppy needs. The bone in raw chicken wings is full of iron containing marrow. This helps build your pup's blood and immune system.

The only nutrients which may be in short supply are some of the B vitamins. However, I have raised large numbers of puppies on raw meaty bones and precious little else. They have done extaordinarily well. Certainly much much better than a pup fed on one of the supposedly complete and balanced top class commercial dog foods.

We choose chicken and chicken bone for another reason. Human health. With chickens as opposed to sheep or beef or pork, there is absolutely no chance of humans getting Hydatids. This fact is of importance to sheep farmers and urban hunters. However, dog owners obtaining sheep, beef and pork products from their butcher have no worries. For more information on Hydatidosis, see Chapter 9.

Chicken bones have another advantage. Because they are derived from very young animals... they contain no toxins, as is possible in bones from old animals. Another benefit of them having come from young animals is that the bones are soft and easy for a puppy to chew. Also, chicken wings are just the right size for small animals... manageable. They are also the right size for an animal that may have to eat in the house... they seem in our experience to be less trouble.. and the puppy always eats the lot ... all gone .. no problems.

The bottom line is that raw chicken wings and necks are fantastic nutrition for your puppy. Meaty lamb bones are almost as good .. but not lamb shanks too often. The bone in lamb shanks is too hard for puppies. Some people feed shank bones to very young pups.... this can be a problem because all the pups get is the meat, they cannot chew up these very hard bones.

It is Absolutely Essential that Young Puppies Actually Eat the Bones

- One of the most important group of nutrients puppies derive from bones are their mineral requirements. This is a point I really want to emphasise, particularly in relation to their calcium needs.

So many people, when they raise puppies, particularly the giant breeds, make mistakes with calcium supplementation. This is because trying to juggle various foods and various calcium supplements to obtain the correct ratio and amount of calcium and phosphorus is an almost impossible task.

It is also a major headache for any one trying to advise you. This does not have to be. The answer to this particular headache is so simple.....

Bones supply your puppy with it's complete mineral requirements in perfect amount and perfect balance. There is no need for calcium supplements when you feed bones.

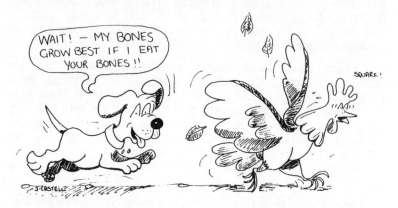

Calcium supplements given to a bone eating puppy are not only unnecessary, they will cause problems... bone problems. Nor do you have to worry about giving too many raw meaty bones.

- Raw meaty bones are not like calcium supplements where the amount to give is critical, and in most cases almost impossible to figure. The simple rule of thumb is to ensure that your puppy receives about sixty percent of it's diet as raw meaty bones.
- It is because this method is so simple, many people refuse to believe it or do it ! They seem to think that because calcium supplementation of pups has always been a headache, feeding bones is just too good to be true.

Dental Health

If you have read the chapters on bone eating, you will know that when your puppy eats bones, it is getting it's teeth cleaned and it's gums massaged.

- Teeth of young puppies cannot grow strong and become firmly embedded in the skull if they are not stressed by bone eating when the puppy is young and developing.

Dogs that eat raw meaty bones as a young pup and continue this practise into adulthood, never develop tartar, and very rarely develop dental problems. This saves the dog a lot of pain and ill health, helps promote a long life, and saves the owner of that dog a lot of money.

Many people want to believe that nylon bones are good for their puppy's teeth. I suppose they might be if the puppy chewed on them, but where is the joy for a dog chewing a nylon bone ? It is like chewing gum long after the flavour has gone. There is no incentive other than destructiveness or boredom in chewing on a nylon bone, and no other virtue beyond teeth cleaning. Nylon bones are a great way to produce a bowel blockage.

- Similarly, dry dog foods do not clean teeth and they are awful nutritionally.

Eating Exercise

One vital form of exercise, mostly denied the modern puppy, is the exercise derived from the chewing of raw meaty bones, particularly the larger bones.

The exercise resulting from bone eating perfectly stresses every one of a puppy's bones, and beautifully tones practically every muscle in it's body. Watch a puppy eating a bone and you will know what I mean.

Picture that puppy, both front paws planted firmly on it's bone, shoulders braced, back legs standing firm, then head down and rip and tear away. That puppy is working it's jaws, neck, shoulders, front legs, back and hind legs. It is using practically every muscle, joint and bone in it's body.

Eating this way helps produces perfect angulation of bones, and strong healthy muscles. This is quite apart from the beneficial effect that bone eating has on teeth and gums.

Compare this daily exercise of ripping and tearing and chewing bones, with a commercial dog food puppy that sucks down a plateful of slop, or a bowl of biscuits, or mince. Head down, a few quick gulps and the food is gone. No exercise of any muscle in the body. No teeth cleaned, just a belly full of lifeless food. Food that sits as a leaden lump in a swollen flabby belly of a thinly muscled pup that will never grow to it's full potential.

I constantly see such pups brought into the surgery. They have not, cannot and do not develop their body to anything like the level of excellence of a bone eating puppy. Bone eating pups, if compared to commercially fed pups, will be found to have much more developed and defined muscles. [See P. 125]

This whole body exercising seen with bone eating, is actually a form of isometric exercise. Exercise where the muscles remain under tension. One of the many benefits of this type of exercise is that it helps in the vital role of keeping the hips tight in larger dogs prone to hip dysplasia. Strong muscles round the hip joint are highly correlated with freedom from hip dysplasia. This is another benefit not available to the commercially fed dog.

- In other words, quite apart from the incredibly high nutritional value of bones to growing dogs, dogs that eat bones regularly while they are growing will be far less likely to develop bone problems because of the continual and vital exercise bone eating forces them to engage in.

Sheer Joy

Eating bones for a dog is a joyous experience. It is so enjoyed by dogs that it actually of itself boosts their immune system.

Meaty Bones make Puppy Owners Lazy... but it's OK !

We have found that we can get away with feeding puppies almost one hundred percent chicken wings, chicken necks and lamb off cuts and very little of anything else. The pups I speak of here are some of our rescue jobs. Crossbreed pups brought in to our hospital for various reasons over the years. Puppies we take pity on.. get them going... and find them a home.

Living where we do, these pups always have access to soil and cow poop. These two "foods" probably contain the nutrients which may be missing from the bones. That is, they provide some of the B vitamins and iodine and essential fatty acids. On the other hand we had similar success when we lived in the city, where they had no access to either cow droppings or soil !

Of course I am speaking about our laziness here. We often do not have a lot of time to be fiddling about with these pups.

- That is how we came to discover just how easy this puppy raising business is. That is how we came to discover that regular feeding is not necessary. That you can produce healthy dogs from very weedy and sickly pups as long as you feed lots of raw meaty bones, with occasional other things such as porridge meals, household scraps, brewer's yeast, kelp and olive or safflower oil.

However, I am getting a bit ahead of myself. I hope by now you believe me when I tell you, firstly how EASY it is to raise puppies successfully using raw meaty bones as the basis of their diet, and secondly how IMPORTANT it is that you do decide to feed your puppies that way.

Before Your Puppy Arrives

Go shopping and buy some chicken wings, brewer's yeast, kelp tablets or powder, some quick cooking rolled oats, some eggs, some canola oil, and some safflower oil. Buy a cleaver and/ or a meat mallet. Have a litle bit of minced meat on hand. Have some fresh green veggies on hand.

- That is your puppy starter kit.

I am assuming your puppy is about six to eight weeks old, and is in good health. I do not have a clue what your pup has eaten up until now, but I am assuming it is eating solids.

Let me assume you have followed my advice. You have brought your puppy home and not over fed it. Your puppy is now hungry.

- Offer your puppy a little bit of minced meat. Beef, lamb, pork, chicken... it doesn't matter. Not totally lean, not too fatty. .... WOOF ! Gone ? Great, excellent. Is your puppy still hungry ? Fine let it be hungry for a moment. You are now going to try it with a chicken wing.

Now lots of puppies will eat a raw chicken wing straight off... no preparation at all. Others, particularly the smaller breeds, or puppies that have only ever eaten sloppy foods, find it difficult to get the hang of being a dog... that is, eating chicken wings.. at first.

To get those overly humanised puppies started, you often have to cut into the chicken a little bit, to expose the flesh. Most hungry puppies, once they have tasted that chicken flesh... grab it out of your hand and get stuck into it.

Some very small, very finicky puppies need even more help. They need you to turn that chicken wing into mince before they will touch it. Remember we did the mince test above.... they ate that very readily.

Turning that chicken wing into mince is why you need a cleaver or a meat mallet in your puppy starter kit. You need a chopping block as well. Take that cleaver or possibly a meat mallet and bash away at that chicken wing until it is all bashed up into a very fine mince... bones and all. Alternatively, use your food processor to mince it up.

If your little puppy will still not eat it... it could be sick, it may not be hungry, it might still be miserable, or if it ate the mince... then it is addicted to mince. If it was a very tiny pup, the mince might have filled it.

If you believe it is still hungry, but that it is addicted to mince, mix the tiniest bit of minced chicken wing with some mince. Every time you feed the mince add a little bit more chicken wing, until in the end, you are feeding pure minced chicken wing.

- This may take three or four days, but it is worth the fiddle. Do not give up and just feed mince... Warning... you will produce a problem puppy if you do ! It will be totally deficient in calcium, iodine and copper etc.. For more information read about the dangers of an all meat diet in Chapter 4.

With the finicky puppies, once you have got them eating the minced chicken wings, you gradually mince it less and less, until in the end, they are eating a whole wing that has not been interfered with at all.

- Your puppy is eating chicken wings ! Great... That means you are well on the way to a healthy puppy.

Feeding Other Things to Balance the Chicken Wings

The principles or secrets of successful puppy rearing which concern us here are firstly number three.. feeding a wide variety of foods... remember, your puppy being an omnivore can eat anything and it is important to accustom it to eat as many different sorts of food as possible. Secondly number four.. feed mostly raw foods, and number nine.. balance that diet over time and do not try and balance up every meal.

- To get you thinking about what else you could or should feed your puppy, focus your mind on the various food groups other than meat and meaty bones such as the fruit and vegetable foods, the grain and legume foods, protein foods such as eggs, the dairy foods, the offal foods and the food supplements.

-

These are all perfectly acceptable foods to feed your puppy. They are all capable of supplying your puppy with nutrients for growth.

The Porridge Meal Recipe

First of all, let's talk about adding grains to your puppy's diet. That is why I got you to buy some rolled oats in the starter kit. If you read the chapter on grains, you will see that rolled oats are a suitable food for puppies, in fact for dogs of all ages.. as an addition to the basic bone diet. But not in large amounts.

Use the quick cooking ones because they have been broken up into very small pieces. This makes it easier for your puppy to digest them

The oats are best cooked up into porridge in the usual way or alternatively you may soak them for an hour or so, or even over night. This is equally as good. preferably feed them at body temperature. They should end up being a nice mushy consistency.

- To a cup of this prepared oatmeal porridge [cooked or soaked], add a teaspoon or two of of honey, a teaspoon of olive oil, a teaspoon of brewer's yeast, several dessert spoons of suitably prepared vegetables [crushed, pulverised etc.], some dried fruit, some shredded coconut, and half a crushed kelp tablet. You could add an egg or an egg yolk or two. We often do, even though it is not consistent with the idea of separating starch and protein meals.

What have you got ? You have got a high energy, high fibre, high vitamin food. Not a complete food.... because the minerals and the protein are missing, or if you did add an egg, just the minerals are missing.

- This does not matter. The minerals will come from the chicken wings you are feeding at other meals. You can quite happily feed this sort of food once a day, or once every second day.

Other meals which you can feed to balance out the chicken wings include vegetable meals, milk, egg and honey meals, straight meat meals, and once or twice a week, a meal containing liver or kidneys or brains etc..

Note That No Meal is Ever Complete and Balanced.

In other words, you should never attempt to make each meal a complete and balanced one. So long as there is a balance of nutrients over a period of about three to seven days that is fine. There is no harm of course if a meal is "complete and balanced" occasionally, but not all the time.

- The more different foods you feed your puppy, the better he or she will be.

The Vegetable Meal

If you have not already done so, read the chapters on vegetables and raw foods. Done that ? .. Good... you now know that the best way to feed your puppy vegetables is to put raw vegetables through the juicer and then recombine the pulp and the juice.

Recipe

Into a cup of this vegetable pulp/mush, you can throw a beaten egg, the brewer's yeast, the kelp powder and the olive oil. If it is winter, use cod liver oil once a week. If for some reason you cannot do the vegetables that way, then half lightly steamed and mashed, mixed with half raw and pulverised is a good way to get puppy started. So is hunger.

By adding egg, you are ensuring your pup obtains an excellent supply of first class amino acids, and some essential fatty acids, and plenty of healthy vitamin A. and D.

If you like, for a change, to either the porridge or the vegetables, instead of egg, or as well as egg, you might like to throw in some offal such as liver or some dairy foods. A heaped tablespoon of yoghurt, or grated cheese, or cottage cheese. All excellent growth foods for our little puppy.

- You may also feed table scraps to your puppy. so long as they are good healthy sorts of growth foods. For more information on feeding table scraps see Chapters 4 and 15.

WARNING

Keep in mind that these other meals are fine, but make sure that the bulk of your puppies diet.. at least half, and preferably –

- 60 % - 80 % .... is raw meaty bones !

How Much Food Should I Feed my Puppy ?

- This question involves principle or secret number two. That is, the importance of keeping puppies lean and not growing them at maximum growth rate. Fortunately with this question, there are some simple rules of thumb.

The first rule of thumb is that up to three months of age, feed three to four meals a day. From three to six months of age feed two to three meals a day, from six to twelve months feed two meals a day, and after twelve months of age, feed one meal a day.

The second rule of thumb is that at each meal, let the pup eat as much as it is able to in ten minutes. After that, take the food away. This guideline is really only appropriate when feeding something like dry dog food.

However, neither are bad guidelines. They have evolved from the experience of countless puppy owners over the years. Despite that, they must be combined with the important guidelines we have already discussed.

- The idea of always leaving your puppy a little bit hungry.
- Not growing your puppy at maximum growth rate.
- Occasionally, say once or twice a week, fast your puppy on fluids only for twelve hours.
- Do not allow your puppy to become fat and roly poly.
- Keep your puppy slim, active and athletic.

In other words, the bottom line is...

- Learn to look at your pup.
- If you are not sure whether it is too fat, too thin or just right, then check with your vet.

Don't Be a Slave to Rules !

When it comes to two, three or four meals a day.. please do not be a slave to that. They are a very rough guide only. It is not vital that your puppy be fed like clockwork.. i.e. always three or four times a day, and at the same time.

- I think it is a great idea to vary the time when your puppy gets fed. It may suit you to feed your puppy on a rigid schedule..... if so fine go for it, but if it just as convenient and suits your lifestyle and working schedule to feed your puppy at odd times... then go for that.

Eating at irregular times is the way both puppies and adult dogs eat under natural conditions. They eat when they are hungry, and when the food becomes available.

- I believe it is important that not all demands made by your puppy are met.. That is, as and when your puppy wants them. In other words, while I do not advocate strict timetable feeding, neither do I recommend demand feeding. It should be a combination of puppy being hungry, and what suits you... the owner.

So feed ... when puppy is hungry, definitely not on schedule, and not necessarily just when puppy says he or she is ready. In fact, let those times when it is actually difficult for you to get home and feed your puppy be that time when you give your puppy a very healthy fast.

- You have to temper the idea of not growing your puppy too fast with it's opposite... not producing stunting and starvation. This is common sense stuff. In other words, severe food restriction will result in permanent damage to your pup. If we could put a figure on it, you should feed your pup about three quarters of what it would eat were it allowed to eat as much as it wanted.

There is No Scientific Formula to Help You

What I cannot do is give you a set of figures which tells you how much food should be fed for a given weight and age of pup. That does not work. There are too many variables. You are going to have to learn to look at your dog critically and use your common sense.

- Your puppy should obviously be growing... that is why, when your puppy arrives, weigh it. Weigh it every week, and keep a record of your puppy's weight.

Another rule of thumb is that you should be able to easily feel your puppy's ribs, but you should not be able to see them. Of course that rule refers to a short haired dog. You will have to part the hair of your long haired dog, or examine it when it is soaking wet.

Let me repeat. If in doubt about whether your puppy is growing at an acceptable rate, that is, whether it is growing too fast and too fat, or whether it is growing too slow, too thin and too held back, or whether it is just right........ check with your vet.

Vitamin Supplements for Pups

If you have no idea at all about this subject please refer to Chapter 5. In that chapter I spoke about the five possible levels of vitamin content in food.

Very briefly, these were.. first level.. not enough, second level.. just enough to prevent severe deficiency symptoms, third level.. vitamins in abundance, that is sufficient extra vitamins to cover most stresses, fourth level, vitamins at pharmacologic levels.. the levels where vitamins can be used like drugs in treating a wide range of disorders, and the fifth or toxic level.

The important point is that sensible supplementation will never do any harm. It makes up for any deficiencies in the diet. That is, adding vitamins to your puppy's diet so that they reach that third level of "vitamins in abundance" is a great idea. On the other hand, excessive supplementation of vitamins like vitamin A and vitamin D can, if taken to extremes [the fifth level], be toxic and therefore cause problems.

- Where it was once thought most vitamins were only necessary in pretty small amounts [the second level], modern research is showing that many of them have roles we have not known about.... roles involved in preventing degeneration and ageing. In these roles, they are not only tolerated in larger amounts, the body actually requires them in larger amounts than previously thought. The third to fourth levels.

The B Complex Group

For puppies, a balanced supplement of B vitamins daily will never cause a problem.

Any excesses will be removed by your pup's kidneys. Your pup simply piddles them out.

- In other words, even if your puppy's diet is supplying adequate B vitamins, supplying extra will do no harm. As a guide, for large puppies, feed a child's dose, and for small puppies, half a child's dose daily.

Vitamin C

Vitamin C is the safest and least toxic vitamin known. In the wild, because dogs eat a lot of raw vegetable material, they are supplied in their diet with large amounts of vitamin C. In addition, because they are on a healthier diet, their liver actually manufactures more vitamin C than a modern dog eating cooked home made or commercial diets.

Daily supplementation of vitamin C has in our experience only ever produced good results. As a guide, 500 mg of vitamin C with each meal is fine, and more can only do good. In fact, vitamin C can be added to the point where it will cause diarrhoea, then back off a bit. That would then be regarded as the maximum dose. For maximum benefit, vitamin C should be given several times a day. This is only necessary however, when the vitamin C is being used to treat an acute problem, such as if your puppy was developing a bone problem.

The Fat Soluble Vitamins:

Vitamins A and D, can be supplied for your puppy by giving a teaspoon of cod liver oil once a week.

Vitamin E can be supplied as a supplement... vitamin E capsules. For an average sized puppy, 200 mg [i.u.] daily. Vitamin K is both manufactured by your puppy in its intestines in adequate amounts, and is a vitamin that is found everywhere in fresh green leafy foods.

Play is Ideal Exercise for Growing Dogs

For a puppy, play is the preferred type of exercise. It is controlled exercise. The puppy controls it, because the puppy determines when enough is enough. The puppy will stop playing when it gets tired or sore. It is normal, natural, and is positively healthful. Indeed it is essential.

- In play, a puppy stops exercising before any damage to it's bones or joints occurs. When puppies are forced to take part in long boring walks, they often continue long after damage has begun to occur to their joints. This is the origin of many problems later in life including hip dysplasia and other skeletal problems such as arthritis.

Why Not Feed Dog Food to our Pup and be Done with It ?

- In fact that is the suggestion and strong advice of many vets. So is it a good idea or a bad idea ?

What your vet means when he gives you that advice, is that you should seek out and find the PERFECT PUPPY GROWING FOOD.

What you will be looking for, is a first rate commercial puppy food, balanced perfectly for all nutrients, no excesses, no deficiencies. It will contain between 1.0% and 2.0% calcium. No more and no less.

The phosphorus in that food will also be between 1.0 % and 2.0 %, but will always be slightly less than the calcium.

It will have the perfect amount of protein for growth, and that protein will be of the highest possible quality. It will have the perfect amount of fat with a perfect balance of essential fatty acids.

It will be perfectly balanced for all minerals which will be in a perfectly available form.

That food will have all vitamins in abundance, but none at the toxic levels.

- Find that perfect puppy food is the advice given by the veterinary profession, feed only that with no supplements and your puppy will have the best chance of growing normally.

Those vets are quite correct. If their clients follow that advice, they will almost certainly have very healthy puppies... to a point. For example, all the benefits of bones would be missing.

That means poor dental health for a start.

- There is another problem with that advice. For the Australian consumer, such a commercial dog food does not exist. Even if it did, it would be impossible to find, because nobody has done the appropriate trials which would tell us which one it is.

There are no puppy foods marketed in Australia with a guarantee that the optimum levels of calcium and other nutrients have been added.

However, even if you could find such a product, that guarantee means nothing unless those foods have been extensively and exhaustively tested by independent authorities.

In other words, there are no commercial puppy foods in Australia which have been shown to do a perfect job of raising puppies in scientifically controlled trials. Trials involving comparisons with a properly formulated, whole, raw-food diet.

- All products currently available in Australia fall far short of those exacting standards.

You could say, let's forget about all that, and simply rely on the claims of the companies. In fact most modern dog owners do precisely that. They have this mistaken belief that commercial dog foods are the best way to feed dogs. They believe the advertising put out by the dog food companies.

Unfortunately, all those claims which the dog food producers either make or allude to, are not supported by properly conducted trials on large numbers of litters of puppies. It is all advertising hype. Masses of empty words, hot air, designed by advertising executives who have been paid lots of money to get people to buy the product.

If you think about it, and face to face in my surgery, so many people realise the truth of this, advertisers will say anything which they can get away with, to sell their product to a gullible public. A public willing to put on their rose coloured glasses and believe anything they are told about dog food... because they want to believe it... for the sake of convenience.

- Let me stress that as a vet, I see the numerous problems on a daily basis that occur when commercial dog food is the only source of nutrients fed to puppies. For more information on the problems inherent in commercial dog foods, refer to Chapter 3.

You might now be asking.. what about all the different diets put out by dog breeders ?

I have never yet come across a good one. One based on the principles discussed in this chapter. In fact I could probably fill an entire book, talking about all the different diets that breeders advocate and that people use to rear puppies. We could pull these diets apart, analyse them, discuss the merits and demerits of each, and show how each of them could be corrected to produce a diet which is reasonable to fair. But what would be the point.

- All you need do, is feed your puppy using the simple and commonsense principles I have described, and all will be well.

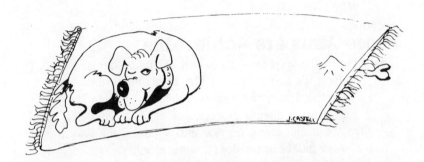

18

Feeding the Adult Dog

LET'S AIM AT SOMETHING !

The first thing I want to discuss with you are the goals or objectives of feeding your adult dog. They are pretty simple really.

- GOAL NUMBER ONE is brilliant health ... both short and long term.

Short term, no dental problems, no skin problems, no ear problems, no eye problems, no bowel problems, in fact no health problems of any description plus a dog that is full of energy, bright, alert, active etc..

Long term, this healthy state should continue into advanced old age without any major disease problems. That is, no heart disease, no kidney disease, no diabetes or arthritis etc.. Dental health should also continue into old age. Poor dental health goes hand in hand with poor general health.

- GOAL NUMBER TWO is that your dog should maintain a steady weight, throughout it's life. That is, it's ideal weight. This will be achieved through a combination of eating and exercise.

Those Aims are Achievable.

- To maximise your dog's health, including dental health, to prolong it's active healthy life, to maintain ideal body weight and minimise health problems including the degenerative disease processes of old age, your dog should be fed a diet based on raw meaty bones, the way it always has been for dogs.... until recently.
- In addition, you should consider the addition of extra vitamins, particularly the anti-oxidant vitamins A, C and E, together with B complex, particularly B1, B5 and B6.

FEEDING DOGS IS SO EASY !

As I stated in the introduction, this book should consist of about three lines. Those lines would read as follows............

- "If you feed your dog on a diet consisting of about 60 % raw meaty bones, with the rest being made up of good quality human food scraps... you will have a healthy trouble free dog. "

Those few words embody all of the principles I have outlined earlier in the book. That is......

Principle Number One

- The bulk of your dog's diet should be raw meaty bones.

Those raw bones with meat supply the bulk of your dog's dietary needs, including it's energy requirements, it's protein requirements, it's mineral requirements [and that includes all the calcium it needs], and if the meat and bones are derived from chickens, most of it's essential fatty acid requirements. Great stuff !

Bones have many other benefits of course, including most importantly........ dental health.

Principle Number Two...

- Feed your dog a wide variety of foods, based on the type and quantity of foods a wild dog would eat.

That is, lots of green vegetables [to mimic stomach contents of prey], some offal, [liver, kidneys etc.], meat, eggs, milk, brewer's yeast, yoghurt and small amounts of grains and legumes... etc..

The important point to remember is that apart from raw meaty bones, no other single food item should ever become the main part of your dog's diet.

Principle Number Three

- Most of your dog's food should be raw.

Principle Number Four

- Your dog should have a balanced diet over all, but not every meal needs to be balanced. Balance is better achieved over time, during the consumption of lots of different meals.

Principle Number Five

- Watch your dog and vary it's diet accordingly.

This mostly refers to it's weight. If your dog is becoming too heavy, you must feed it less food, less energy-rich food and you must feed it less frequently. It also refers to more subtle indicators of health such as the state of the coat. For example a dry lustreless coat would indicate that not enough essential fatty acids were being fed, and you would increase eggs or chicken or oil etc. accordingly.

Healthy Meals for Your dog

The nutrients not supplied by raw meaty bones include some vitamins, all carbohydrate requirements, [iodine ?], fibre, maybe some essential fatty acids and probably some longevity factors.

You are going to balance that basically raw meaty bone diet using foods which are mostly of plant origin, plus small amounts of offal, eggs, vegetable oils and dairy foods etc..

Green leafy vegetables should make up about 60 % - 70 % of the vegetable part of the diet, with grain and starchy vegetables being between 20 % - 30 %. The offal portion of the diet, that is, liver, kidneys and hearts etc. should be about 5.0 % - 15 % of the diet. Throw in some eggs two or three times a week. More often if you wish.

To help you understand how to do this, I am going to describe a series of simple meals which can be quickly and easily prepared and fed to your dog. These meals are based on the principles which we have been talking about, including food separation and combination. They are meal ideas which you can use to balance up a diet based on mostly raw meaty bones.

I include first of all, the food list that was developed in Chapter 5. Use this list as a jog to your memory when preparing meals for your dog.

Animal Products

Raw meaty bones from chicken, lamb, beef, rabbit, pork.

Muscle meat from chicken, lamb, beef, pork

Organ meat - liver, kidneys, heart, brains

Eggs, especially the yolk

Cheese and cottage cheese, yoghurt, milk, butter

Seafoods - any fatty fish, herring, salmon, sardines etc.

Plant Products

Fresh, green leafy vegetables such as spinach, outer leaves of lettuce, cauliflower, broccoli, brussel sprouts etc.

Corn, sweet potatoes [the yellow ones], pumpkin, squash

Mushrooms

Root vegetables, potatoes, carrots, radishes, turnips, parsnips
Fresh and dried fruits – any of them

Legumes – peas and beans, baked beans etc

Whole grains including brown rice and oat flakes, wheat
germ, wheat bran, wholemeal bread

Miscellaneous

Brewer's yeast, kelp powder or tablets, molasses.

Oils

Cod liver oil, corn oil, soyabean oil, wheat germ oil, cottonseed oil, safflower oil, sunflower oil, peanut oil

RECIPES

The Green Leafy Vegetable Meal

Remember, vegetables are best fed raw. If you are unsure
how raw vegetables should be prepared for dogs, please turn to
Chapter 10.

●   If you need to get your dog used to vegetables, steam
     and mash half of them, and add these to the raw
     pulverised vegetables. Let it cool to body temperature.
     For each cup of vegetables add from half to two whole
     eggs or yolks only, and a teaspoon of oil, and a teaspoon
     of apple cider vinegar, and a teaspoon of brewer's yeast.
     For variation, instead of the egg, add a similar quantity
     of cottage cheese, ordinary cheese, or minced beef, or one
     of the organ meats put through the blender.

Depending on how fat your dog is, you can vary the additives to this meal. If your dog is fat, reduce the additives, especially oil and protein additives. If your dog is too thin, these can
be increased.

The Starchy Meal

This is a basically cooked meal. It will consist of one or more of potatoes, rice, pumpkin, sweet potato, bread, pasta, oats etc.. To this add such things as yoghurt, oil, dried fruits, milk and green leafy vegetables....suitably pulverised, brewer's yeast and kelp.

Cereals are useful to feed in winter, particularly brown rice or oatmeal porridge. Serve it up nice and warm. For extra energy you may add butter or one of the oils. During cold periods, you may have to feed extra food to maintain your dog's weight, particularly if your dog spends a lot of time outdoors, and particularly if it is exercising a lot.

The Grain and legume Meal

These must be cooked of course. Combine approximately equal amounts of a cooked grain such as rice or oats and a legume such as baked beans or a three bean mix, or a soup mix etc.. To this mix can be added pulverised green leafy vegetables, preferably raw, and oil and yoghurt and brewer's yeast and kelp etc..

The Meat Meal

As the name suggests, this is where you feed mainly meat. This will happen when you feed a large joint of meat on the bone, or a huge chunk of meat without the bone. It will also happen when you feed minced meat.

This meal can therefore consist of any of the meats you wish. Beef, chicken, lamb, veal, horse, kangaroo etc..

If it is minced, and your dog is not used to eating a lot of offal, mince the offal through this meal. You can also add some or all of egg, fish, cottage cheese, vegetables, oil, brewer's yeast, and kelp.

The Milk "Meal"

This "meal" consists of ordinary cow's milk, about a cup, to which you add two or three egg yolks, or whole eggs if your dog can tolerate them [most dogs can], 5 to 10 ml of one of the vegetable oils, e.g. canola, or safflower or soybean or corn oil etc., one or two teaspoons of brewer's yeast, and a pinch of "lite" salt.

The Offal Meal

This meal will consist of one or more of such items as liver, kidney, heart, brain tripe etc.. Many butchers will prepare a mix of this nature and label it "dog's delight". Many dogs can eat an all offal meal with no problems. Others will refuse to eat it, yet others will throw up afterwards.

Offal is important for your dog, containing as it does, many different nutrients including essential vitamins and minerals.

If your dog has difficulty eating offal, start off with a small amount mixed in with one of the other meals, such as the minced meat meal, the green leafy vegetable meal, or even the milk and egg meal .. after it has been put through the blender.

The Food Scraps Meal

The ideal way to approach any food scraps you may have is to decide into which of the above categories they fit. The only reason you will do that is because having made that decision, you can more intelligently balance youir dog's diet [over time of course], in accordance with the section on balance which you are about to read.

It is also worthwhile reading Chapter 15 for more information on food scraps as part of your dog's diet.

Achieving Balance

This is absurdly easy.

- A balanced diet for your dog would consist of approximately 10 bone meals combined with 4 green leafy vegetable meals, 1 starchy meal, 1 grain and legume meal, 1 purely meat meal, 2 milk meals and 1 or 2 offal meals. This would occur over a 2 to 3 week period.

The other way some of you may want to approach this question of balance is in terms of protein, carbohydrates, fats, minerals and vitamins etc. That is, ideally you will wish to supply adequate quantities of all of these in terms of the essential amino acids, the essential fatty acids, together with the correct balance and amounts of all the different vitamins and minerals.

- That is the academic approach and very commendable, but also practically impossible.

Unfortunately, we still do not know exactly what a dog's requirements are in those terms. However, there is no need to worry. If you feed your dog as I have just described then it is impossible not to supply all those necessary nutrients for your dog. Not only that, you will also supply nutrients necessary for your dog's health which you don't know about !

- NOTE: If your dog is obese, feed lots and lots of veggies, in place of grain and meat.... particularly feed the less starchy more leafy vegetables. Lots of raw carrot is fine. So is fruit.

Once More in a Nutshell

- To put all that in very simple terms, lots of raw meaty bones, fed almost every day, lots of green leafy vegetables, small amounts of grain and starch type products, some eggs, some oil, some dairy foods, and about once a week throw in some offal products. Daily or several times a week add such things as brewer's yeast and kelp.

GENERAL NOTES ON FEEDING YOUR DOG THIS WAY

Do Feed Different Types of Raw Meaty Bones.

That is, chicken, lamb, beef and even pork if it is not too dear. We feed about 60 % - 70 % chicken, the remainder being lamb, rabbit, beef, pork or whatever. The reason for the higher levels of chicken is partly because of availability, and partly because of the better levels of essential fatty acids in raw meaty chicken bones compared to other meaty bones.

- If other bones are more available where you live such as beef and/or lamb, use those. If you cannot get a lot of chicken bones, you may have to add extra oil to give your dog adequate essential fatty acids.

The bones available will vary as to the amount of meat on them. For example, if feeding whole chickens, or legs of lamb, you may be feeding lots more meat than bone.

It is better to reduce the meat in most instances. For example, two parts of meat to one part of bone, or more frequently three or four parts bone to one part of meat. Boned out chicken carcases are good in this regard, as are chicken wings, or lamb offcuts from the butcher.

Up to 40 % of the raw meaty bones you buy may be fat. A lot of that fat will be in the bones themselves as invisible fat, but about half of it may be visible fat.

It is often necessary to trim off some or most of that visible fat, particularly with very fatty chicken or with lamb. This will depend on such factors as the weight of the dog, and the amount of work it is doing. The harder your dog works, the more fat it will need to maintain it's body weight. Remember that raw fat is much healthier than cooked fat.

As your dog becomes overweight, it is important to reduce the fat, but pay more attention to a greater concentration of the essential fatty acids. That is, make sure that the fats fed come from chicken and pork fat, or eggs or vegetable oils.

Some dogs simply cannot tolerate very fatty meat. Only your own experience with your own dog will tell you this.

Bone Burying

When your dog proceeds to bury it's bones, take them away. Your dog is not truly hungry. This is not a signal to stop feeding bones. It is a signal that your dog is being fed too much food. Fast your dog for at least twelve hours, and then try the meaty bones once again.

The Vital Question of Vitamins

Try and copy nature by supplying an over abundance of vitamins in your dog's diet. If you are unsure about. vitamins, please refer to the section on vitamins in Chapter 5.

An excellent source of B vitamins is brewer's yeast. For a healthy 25 kg dog, feed 1 to 3 teaspoons of brewer's yeast daily. If your dog has never had brewer's yeast before start off with half a teaspoon and work up. Remember brewer's yeast is a very concentrated food. Mix it into a suitable meal or dust the powder over the moist raw meat. Not thickly... otherwise it just gets shaken off. [Read about brewer's yeast in Chapter 16.]

If your dog rejects food with brewer's yeast in it, do not just toss the whole idea away as so many people do.

Enlist the aid of hunger. A day or two without food will work wonders, and instead of a huge amount of brewer's yeast, start off with a really tiny amount.. a pinch, one that the dog will never notice, then gradually build it up. All it requires is patience. You will get away with it, to the great benefit of your dog. For a full discussion of brewers yeast see Chapter 16.

Note that you can use this method to get your older dog used to eating anything. If your dog is young, encourage it to eat a wide range of foods, and you will never have this problem.

By feeding liver on a regular basis, you will ensure plenty of the fat soluble vitamins, particularly vitamin A, as well as many of the B vitamins.

If you want to be sure your dog is receiving a super abundance of healthy vitamins, just as a dog in the wild would, you

can supply extra amounts of them as vitamin tablets or capsules.
Extra B's and C can only do your dog good. You may use
"human" vitamins or ones packaged specifically for animals.
Quite often the human ones are cheaper.

● Vitamins may be purchased from your vet, your pet shop,
your health food store, your chemist or by mail order.

If you want your dog to have a super abundant quantity of
vitamin C, use a supplement. Some of it will also come from the
fresh fruit and veggies you will be feeding. Also remember that
the better the rest of the diet, the more vitamin C your dog will
make for itself.

As far as the fat soluble vitamins go, most dogs will benefit
from a carefully controlled supplement of vitamin A and plenty
of vitamin E. Extra D will be required by dogs which do not get
a lot of sunlight.. for whatever reason. For example in winter,
add one to two teaspoons of cod liver oil once a week. This will
supply both A and D. You can also feed any offal meats such
as liver, hearts, brains, kidneys etc. once a week. These can be
fed whole or cut up fine or minced and mixed in with other
foods.

If your dog eats plenty of green leafy vegetables and/or liver,
then vitamin K will be in abundance. A faeces eating dog also
gets plenty of vitamin K, as well as all the B vitamins.

Iodine is Essential

To supply iodine, add some kelp tablets daily. For a 25 kg
dog, you can give one a day, or one several times a week. They
are best crushed and mixed in with a suitable meal. If you have
difficulty getting your dog to accept them, do as for brewer's
yeast..... starting off with a tiny amount and building up. Let me
repeat.. do not just give up.

Kelp will also supply other trace minerals. Other sources of
iodine include fish and dairy products. Vegetables may or may
not contain iodine, it all depends on the soil in which they were
grown.

Do not be tempted to use iodised salt to add iodine to your
dog's food.. well not on a regular basis or in large amounts
anyway. The ingestion of huge amounts of salt can cause just
as many heart and kidney problems in dogs as it does in humans.

Longevity Factors

- Keep in mind always, that the greater the variety of fresh whole unprocessed foods you feed to your dog, and the more such foods come to make up the bulk of your dog's diet, the more vitamins and other longevity nutrients your dog will be getting.

The longevity factors are supplied by any and all of the raw foods you are feeding, and also by supplementing with vitamins and brewer's yeast. For longevity always consider supplementing with the vitamins A, C, and E, together with zinc, selenium and the multi B vitamins. Your vet can supply you with selenium tablets.

- Do not be tempted to supply extra calcium . By feeding plenty of bones, you have catered for your dog's calcium and other mineral needs perfectly.

Feeding Lots of Polyunsaturated Oils - Caution

If feeding lots of these to improve your dog's intake of essential fatty acids, it is most important to add extra anti-oxidant type vitamins, especially vitamin E.

Fitting in With the Family

In the Mornings

If it is your habit to feed the family a cereal meal, let the dog have the same. Of course I don't mean one of those horrible sugar filled processed cereals... not at all... I mean oat meal... or some other whole grain porridge. Prepare it the night before by soaking the oat meal in water or milk... If using milk, then preferably raw. E.g. goat's milk is available raw.

Add honey, yoghurt, dried fruit such as raisins or sultanas, dessicated coconut, sesame seeds or tahini etc..

On the other hand, you may elect to feed your dog his or her raw meaty bones in the morning. This will give your dog something to do all day. In this case you could make your dog's evening meal similar to your own. That is of course if you are feeding your dog two meals on that day.

In the Evenings

If your family is having meat and vegetables, consider a similar meal for the dog. It does not have to be exactly the same as your meal. For instance, you will not cook it!

A meat only meal is fine occasionally. You might choose that particular night to add some organ meat to your dog's food. Some dogs love organ meat and will eat it with no coaxing whatsoever. Others will need it minced and mixed through other minced foods.

Having a Barbeque ?

You may elect to feed meat only on a night you are having a barbecue. Preferably raw of course. Yes, I know your dog will get the cooked left overs. Like anything else.. a little bit of what you fancy does you good.

- There is absolutely nothing wrong with feeding a few cooked meat scraps to your dog.... occasionally.
  Remember, it is what you do most of the time that makes the difference.

WARNING... Don't forget that cooked bones can be very dangerous. I have seen dogs with their insides impaled on sharp T bones or clogged up with "bone cement" after a huge barbecue where all the participants simply threw their left over bones to the dogs. So educate the children AND the guests !

Mincing Helps

If you decide to feed your dog a mainly green leafy vegetable meal, and this is a new idea for your dog, add a little bit of minced meat to the vegetables to make sure your dog eats them. In this case, both the meat and veggies should be so finely minced and mixed that your dog cannot separate them out. Some dogs are expert at this.

The other advantage of fine mincing means that the meat taste permeates the veggies. It is a natural thing to do, because the dogs love the minced up veggies found in their prey's intestines. On subsequent similar occasions, simply add less meat until your dog is enjoying pure veggies. Remember, the choices as with your own food are endless.

Speaking of vegetables, you do not have to use the very best for your dog. You can visit your local fruit and vegetable shop, and pick up the rubbish bits that would normally be tossed away. These are usually available for nothing. Also, all the vegetable peelings from the preparation of the family's food may be minced up for the dog.... use what ever you have. The peels do in fact hold most of the nutrients. Preferably feed them raw. [see chapter 10 for details on preparing raw veggies for your dog.]

WARNING... The only factor which would stop you feeding these outer leaves of vegetables etc. is IF they have been sprayed with chemicals such as insecticides, fungicides, herbicides etc..

Be Flexible

- Something I want to make quite clear is that you do not have to be a slave to any of the above. Do not wander around feeling guilty if what you are doing is not perfect. It never can be. It is important to maintain a relaxed attitude about all of this and be flexible.

It is what you do over a long period of time that counts. It will depend on availability, what you have in the freezer etc.. One week you might feed bones only twice a week, while another week, you might feed meaty bones every day. Sometimes you may have to feed more grains than is ideal. At other times, your dog might go for weeks without them.

- Be flexible, but never get into a lazy rut of feeding only one thing, and never loose the habit of regular raw meaty bones.

What you actually feed depends not only on what is available, but also on the size of your dog. For example, small breeds of dog will do very well on chicken wings or chicken necks, or part of a lamb breast, or a lamb chop, or part of a rabbit. Larger dogs will eat a whole chicken or a whole rabbit, or a number of pieces of lamb off cuts or even one of the giant beef bones... occasionally. If you need to refresh your memory on bones, turn to Chapter 7.

The Question of a Feeding Routine

- I think it is an excellent idea to get your dog used to a variable feeding regime. Sometimes 1 meal a day, sometimes 2, and sometimes none.

This has several benefits, including your lack of concern about being late home and not having fed the dog[s]. Also, if you happen to run out of food, use that as a very good time to fast your dog for twelve to twenty four hours. Far more healthy than going to the cupboard and taking out that tin or packet of processed food you have been saving for just such a time.

It can be practical and healthy in other ways. For example, if you feed your dog a particularly big meal of meat and bones, it is quite a good idea to follow that up with a fast of at least twenty four hours.

- A number of friends, clients and acquaintances have told me that for maximum health, their dogs are best fed every second or third day, particularly when they are not doing very much in the way of work, activity, exercise etc..

In this regard, it must be stressed they are not being cruel. They are treating their dogs properly. Far more cruel is to over feed a dog and produce obesity and subsequently poor health. Perhaps the most cruel way to do that is with commercial dog food because of the severe ill health it causes.

Many people think it important to get their dog into some sort of routine such as always feeding the dogs at a particular time of day. If that suits your lifestyle fine... go for it.

- Actually, such an artificial regime is quite unnatural for a dog. It also makes YOU a slave to your dog. Not a great idea.

One of the best ways of training a dog is to reward it for behaving the way you want it to. The dog demanding to be fed at a particular time is not the way we like our dogs to behave. If you are flexible with your meal times, you can use meals as an impromptu reward for a training session well executed.

At meal times, it is a great idea to train your dog not to eat until you give permission. Put that bowl of food down, and have the dog sitting waiting for your command to allow him or her to eat. This is just another way of establishing yourself as boss. It makes for a much more pleasant and well mannered pet.

Feeding in Relation to Rest and Exercise

One very important feeding rule is to never feed a large meal before any sort of strenuous exercise. Feeding should occur during the four hour period after exercise, but wait for at least an hour until the dog has cooled down. That latter caution probably only applies with poor quality commercial dog food, but nevertheless, it is not a bad precaution to observe.

On that basis, for the average dog, spending most of the day being active, the main meal, the heavy protein or large starch meal should be given at night, with only a small meal in the morning.

How Much Food Should I Feed My Dog ?

This is a very common question asked of vets. It sounds as though it ought to have a simple answer. It does not. Not only that, it is such an important question that I have given it it's own chapter.. the next one......

- 19 -

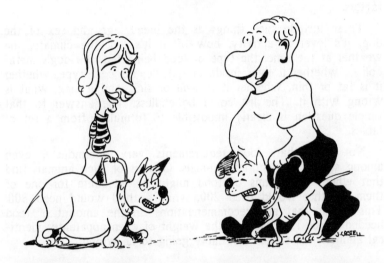

How Much Food do I Feed My Dog and How Often ?

How many times a day should I feed my dog, and how much at each meal ? These are two of the most common questions asked of veterinary surgeons. Unfortunately those questions are impossible to answer in the way that people want them answered. The answers they need - the ones I am about to give you, are simple and practical and useful, but they are not what most people expect.

Firstly - How Much ?

Despite what a lot of people would like to imagine, it is not possible to weigh a dog, consult a set of tables, and then state that it requires X amount of food. There are too many variable factors.

These include such things as the breed, age and sex of the dog, it's level of activity, how often it's fed, the climate, the weather at the time, the type of food being fed, the dog's metabolism, whether it lives inside or outside, it's coat type, whether it is fat or thin, whether it is well or sick, and if sick, what is wrong with it. The list could be endless. The answer to that simple question is clearly impossible to formulate from a set of tables.

Not only that, food requirements vary enormously, even among apparently identical animals. Owners of such animals find that where 100 grams of food might be adequate for one of them, another would need 200, while a third would need 300. This means that any recommendations on the amount of food needed which are based on the weight of even apparently identical animals, are almost invariably going to be wrong.

What About How Often - Can That be Answered ?

Most adult dogs fed with commercial dog foods are fed at least once a day. However, I have found that dogs fed whole raw foods do not crave food the way the commercially fed animal does. They do not require their food to arrive as frequently. They are more satisfied with their food. The dogs fed the commercial product seem to get hungrier sooner after they have eaten.

- That is why an increasing number of dog owners who have started to feed their dogs properly on whole foods are finding they only need to feed their dogs every second or third day.

The dogs in question are magnificiently healthy and happy animals. We commonly, will feed our dogs every second day for a week or so, and then for another week they might be fed daily and then they might have a couple of days fast. It all depends how they are looking, and how much work they are doing.

- But keep in mind, these dogs are being fed fresh, whole foods, not artificial, commercial foods. If you feed a dog that infrequently with artificial foods, because those foods are such poor value, your dog will literally starve. Don't do it !

Do realise that how often and how much are really part of the same question, and the rest of what I have to say involves both. What you will notice is that it all boils down to common sense.

The Rules are Simple !

Despite all that I have said, the process of determining the right amount to feed is very practical and does not involve complicated mathematics. It does involve knowing how to look at a dog and how to weigh a dog, and a general idea of the sorts of foods which are high in calories, and those which are low in calories and rich in fibre.

The Basic Rule

You feed whatever you need to ... to maintain optimum body weight and condition in your dog.... So look at your dog and weigh your dog. Is your dog overweight ? Is your dog underweight. Is your dog just right ? Is your dog gaining weight ? Is your dog losing weight ?

The answer to those questions determines how much food, what type of food, and how often that food should be fed.

Looking at Your Dog

A healthy dog is a slim, athletic creature. It has a light covering of flesh over the ribs. If your dog is getting on in years, and you are not sure how he or she should look, think of what your dog looked like when it was about eighteen months old. Most dogs of that age are at about their ideal weight. If you are not sure, consult your vet.

If your dog is a young adult, and looking good... slim and athletic.. weigh it, record the weight, and strive to keep it at that weight for the rest of it's life by adjusting meal size, content and frequency.

It is Common Sense Really

In other words, if your dog is losing weight, and the cause is not worms or illness etc., then more food more often, should be fed until it reaches it's desired weight and condition. After that, ease back... and adjust meal size and frequency so you keep your dog at that desired weight and condition.

If your dog still does not gain sufficient weight, then food higher in calories must be fed. Usually that means more fat or oil type foods. In some cases, extra protein such as meat and eggs may be required.

If your dog is too heavy, which is a much more common problem, both with the dog and it's master, then you must feed less food less often, and quite often you may have to feed food containing less calories.

Commonly that means substituting meat and fat with lots more fibre-rich vegetables such as carrots, cabbage, spinach etc.. Of course you will also have to consider the question of exercise. Much more of that will be required. let me also stress that it is not necessary to feed your dog every day.

- If you do not adhere to these guidelines, you will find as so many people have in the past, that they have produced a VERY OBESE dog. That dog is then prone to numerous health problems.

- What you have to realise is that in the end there is only one person who can tell you how much and how often your dog should be fed. YOU ! You are the one who must look at your dog, weigh your dog, and adjust meal size and frequency accordingly.

- If it is important to you that your dog receive at least one meal a day, then adjust the size of that meal to ensure no loss or gain of weight - providing it is at it's correct weight already.

Do Not Feed Adult Dogs Like Puppies

A lot of people make the mistake of continuing to feed their young adult dog in the same way they fed it as a puppy. They forget that they were feeding their puppy for growth. Once your dog reaches it's mature size and weight it is important to adjust [reduce] the food intake so as to maintain optimum weight and prevent obesity.

The Exercise Factor

Never forget the exercise factor. Exercise makes an incredible difference. A sedentary dog lying around requires very little food. Not only that, by exercising your dog, you stimulate it's metabolic rate. That is, it burns up energy faster even on those days it is not exercising. As long as you don't exercise your dog out of the window of a car, both of you will be much healthier.

The Influence of Season

During winter, more food is required to keep your dog warm, unless of course it lives inside a heated house all winter.

In summer, because the temperatures are high, and your dog is likely to be lethargic, it will not require as much energy for exercise or to keep it warm. However, despite that, many people find that their dog loses weight in summer. This happens because of two factors. One is a poor appetite which is common in hot weather. The other is that dogs use up an enormous amount of energy keeping cool. They keep cool by panting.

If your dog is over-weight, that summer weight loss is great ! You can help the process along by offering less meat and fat and starchy food in summer or during hot weather. At such times offer fruit and vegetables instead.

However, if your dog is already thin, and losing weight due to a poor appetite in the hot weather, you may actually need to feed very energy-rich food. That is, extra fat or oil, or if the problem is not too severe, may be a bit more starchy food. In this case, it will depend a lot on what your dog finds most appetising. This situation is common with show dogs.

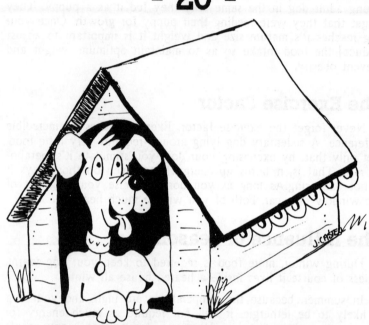

Getting Your Dog Started on It's New Diet

No matter how good a diet is, if your dog will not eat it, it is a complete waste of time, money and effort, and will have no effect on your dog. It is also very frustrating when a dog will not eat something you have gone to a bit of trouble preparing.

It Can be Done !

Lots of people watch their dog deteriorate on it's old cooked and/or commercial dog food diet, simply because they do not know how to persuade it to eat a more healthy diet. This chapter is therefore very important. It is here to teach you how to get even the fussiest dog eating properly.

- Basically, you are going to rely on patience [yours], hunger [your dog's], and low down cunning - [yours].

Many owners simply change their dog's diet. One day the old way, and the next day the new way. No problems, no fuss, no drama. Owners usually know when it will be like this. Their dog is the sort of dog that will "eat anything".

However, this is not always the case. Lots of dogs are very picky when it comes to food. Many have trained their owners as to just exactly what they will and will not eat... almost always to the detriment of their health.

If your dog is like that, refuses to eat the new food, and has you tearing your hair out, or very simply wanting to give it all away because it is much too hard... don't worry. All you need are a few pointers. As usual, it really is very simple.

- There are two basic ways of getting your fussy dog to eat the new food. There is the fasting method and the gradual change method. Then of course, there is the combination of the two.

The fasting method is absurdly simple. All you have to do is not feed your dog for several days until he or she is ready to eat just about anything. In my experience, the only creature this is hard on, is the poor owner. Many owners feel it is their bounden duty to be stuffing food down their dog's throat at every opportunity. When they are not doing that they tend to think they are being cruel and heartless and that their dog will not love them if they did anything different.

WRONG... STOP FEEDING YOUR DOG... You are NOT going to starve your dog. That would be cruel and unnecesary. All you are going to do, is provoke some REAL HUNGER.

- Large numbers of dogs, like ourselves eat way too much food. Many dogs are so over fed, that they often refuse to eat all but a few items to which they have become addicted. In this case, a few days without food will work absolute wonders.

Check With Your Vet Before Fasting Your Dog

- Before you decide to change your dog's diet, do check with your local vet and make sure that should you decide to follow the fasting method, your dog does not have some underlying condition that would make fasting unwise. If your dog is young and healthy, I would not anticipate any problems.

The other method is the GRADUAL CHANGE method. If this is not done properly, it will not work. It is no good adding a few items of fresh whole food to a commercial dog food or some other form of bad feeding to which your dog is addicted. In that case, your dog will simply reject the new foods. At this point a lot of owners give up entirely and go back to their bad feeding habits.

- The trick with a really difficult dog, one that is addicted to just a few food items, is to fool that dog into believing that nothing has changed.
- Step one is to identify that food which your dog absolutely loves.
- Step two is to get your dog used to eating that food in a finely minced state.
- Step three is to finely mince the food you wish to get your dog eating... e.g. a chicken wing.
- Step four is to add a tiny amount of the new food to the much loved minced food. The amount must be so tiny your dog cannot detect it. Hunger helps here. Once your dog is eating this, go to step five.

- Step five is to GRADUALLY INCREASE the amount of the new food in the much loved but minced food. Eventually your dog will be eating the new food by itself. If the new food does not need to be minced, then gradually lessen off the mincing process, until you are feeding it in the form you want it to be fed.

Sometimes a dog will eat part of the new diet, but not other bits. In that case all you have to do, is follow the above steps with the food items it won't eat. For example, many people report that their dog refuses to eat vegetables of any description.

- Do Not Give Up !

Take those vegetables and turn them into mush with a food processor or a juicer. Now go through the process I have just described.

You can win, and your dog will be much happier and healthier and hang around for a much longer time if you can switch it from an unhealthy cooked or processed food diet to a healthy diet based on raw meaty bones.

Many dogs start their new diet with enthusiasm and then suddenly refuse to eat it !

What you have to realise is that when dogs start to eat HEALTHY foods, the dogs you could never fill, the chronically hungry ones will often stop being hungry. For the first time in that dog's life, it is truly satisfied. This will be a new experience for you as well. Such a dog will not be constantly looking for more to eat as it has always done. Understandably, many owners becoming alarmed, thinking their dog is sick.

This often results in an owner ringing me to say... "he really liked those veggies [or whatever] to start with, but for the last couple of nights he has refused to eat them." It's great when they ring and tell me straight away. Then I can reassure them. Tell them to fast their dog for twenty four hours, and then retry either with that sort of natural food or another one in their new repertoire of foods.

Others are so used to their dogs EATING CONSTANTLY, that they find it difficult to disappoint their dogs with foods they don't appear to like. Their dog really has got them by the short and curlies! These folk in an effort to please their dogs and get their dogs to eat something.. resort to feeding them on processed foods once again.

Those foods of course are cooked and have flavour enhancers such as salt. So of course the dog eats them. This often "proves" to the owner that it is actually the old food the dog requires, and the new diet is instantly dropped. DON'T BE FOOLED.

Another way to go at this, particularly with an older dog not used to eating raw food, a dog that has eaten processed food or cooked food all it's life, is to gradually reduce the amount of cooking you do, until eventually, the food is presented in it's raw state.

- By starting your dog on meals that are partly raw and partly cooked, you can gradually get your dog accustomed to eating healthy foods without it being too much of a shock to your dog's system. If changes in diet are made very abruptly, they will sometimes be totally rejected, or if eaten, they may cause diarrhoea.

- 21 -

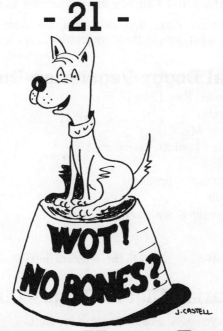

Feeding Your Dog Vegetarian Style

This chapter came into being after I received a letter from a lady who needed information about feeding dogs vegetarian style. The relevant part of her letter went something as follows.....

"What do you know about vegetarian diets for dogs ? I have lots of vegetarian friends with animals that are also vegetarians. People often ask them about vegetarian diets for dogs. They are not one hundred percent sure that they are doing it right. Are they handing out the right advice ?

The following is an outline of the diet used by one of these friends. She has seven rescued mutts. What we would like to know, is this OK ? Can you expand on it ? Can you do better?"

The dietary ideas that lady sent me were very simple, and typical of what people think vegetarian dogs should eat.

Typical Doggy Vegetarian Diet

- Brown Rice [Base]
- Lentils
- Soup Mix
- Salad [carrots, celery etc.]
- Bread
- Vitamin supplement
- Fruit
- Flavoured with vegan gravox

My answer, or at least the relevant bits went as follows.......

Vegetarian Diet for Dogs - Discussion

When you ask about vegetarian diets, I get the impression you mean totally vegetable, with not even the hint of eggs or dairy products or bones ?

- If that is the case, your dogs are missing foods which are vitally important to their health, the most important being raw meaty bones.

Another problem of purely vegetarian diets is the lack of vitamin B12 . Fortunately, you are adding a vitamin supplement. Do check and make sure it contains B12.

A saving factor for a lot of vegetarians is that most vegetables do have some tiny insects left on them, which usually provide this essential vitamin. The other way to provide extra B 12 would be to have your vet give your dog an injection of vitamin B12 once a year with the annual vaccination booster.

Anyway, let me first talk about the good features of the diet you have sent me.

The Good Things About That Diet

- The first good feature is that lentils, a legume, are added to the rice base.

This ensures that the diet is balanced with respect to it's essential amino acids. That is, when a diet includes both legumes and grains, and these are it's major source of proteins, the proteins in this diet will provide a balance of all the essential amino acids.

In those parts of the world where people get most of their protein from vegetable matter, rather than animal sources, they almost always eat a combination of a grain and a legume. Unfortunately, many dog owners are not aware of this.

- The most common mistake is where people feed dogs mostly rice. It is not common to see dogs fed a diet containing mostly legumes, but that would be equally as bad nutritionally, and very "windy".

Both extremes leaves the eater, your dog[s] deficient in some essential amino acids...Over a period of time this can result in a gradual decline in health.

- The second good feature of this diet is that it is a low protein diet. Because this vegetarian diet is low in protein it will promote a long life.

ALL modern nutritional research points the finger at continual excessive protein as a major cause of the degenerative diseases, particularly kidney disease. Low protein is one of the great benefits of a vegetarian diet compared to a meat based diet.

Dogs on high protein diets [i.e. the commercially fed dog] all their life - at every meal, do not last as long as dogs fed restricted amounts of protein or dogs fed a natural diet with varying amounts of protein.

- The third good feature of this diet is that it is a high fibre diet.

This diet contains more than adequate levels of fibre. However, it is mostly cooked fibre. Cooked fibre is much less valuable to the health of dogs than raw fibre. Observations of many hundreds of dogs with the fibre responsive diseases such as obesity and diabetes during eighteen years of practise, shows that they are all less prevalent on a raw diet compared to a cooked diet.

- The fourth good feature is that this is a high potassium diet. That is, having lots of veggies, it is loaded with potassium and low in sodium.

In general, high potassium diets are healthy diets, as opposed to the commercial dog food diets which are high in sodium. The sodium-filled commercial dog foods, actively promote kidney and heart disease.

However, I am not at all sure about the levels of sodium in the vegan gravox.

- Consider substituting the vegan gravox with brewer's yeast, which although high in sodium has many additional nutritional features. Garlic is also an excellent flavouring herb. Use it and other herbs to taste. You also then get the added benefits of the active ingredients in those herbs.

The Bad Things About This Diet

- The first feature that really bothers me about your vegetarian diet apart from the lack of bones is that it is a basically cooked diet.

I am assuming that the rice and lentils form the bulk of this diet. That means many vital nutrients are destroyed before they have a chance to promote the health of your dog. These include many essential vitamins, all the enzymes originally present in the food, plus many naturally occuring anti-oxidants.

It is not so bad in the case of the B vitamins. They are probably being replaced in the added vitamin supplement. However, does your vitamin supplement contain adequate or even any vitamin C ?

Mostly vitamin C has to be added separately. I like to see at least 50 mg per kg per day. On the other hand, there will be some vitamin C in the fruit. The other point is that because your diet is much healthier than most commercial dog food diets, even before you modify it as I suggest, your dogs will in fact be making more vitamin C than the average unhealthy commercially fed dog.

Of course this diet will also contain some enzymes. That is, if the fruit is fresh [not cooked], over-ripe, and there is lots of it. The diet will however be low in naturally occurring anti-oxidants. These are vital in the prevention of degenerative diseases, and the slowing of the ageing process.

- The best way to get around the problem of a lack of anti-oxidants is to add them to the diet. This always makes an incredible difference to the health of dogs. That is, add vitamins A, C, and E in appropriate amounts.

The other way is to make sure that you include absolutely loads of fresh raw foods .. vegetables and fruit .. in the diet.

- The second thing that worries me about many vegetarian dogs is that their diet is mostly rice.

Grains are not a natural food for a dog and will eventually cause problems. There are a number of reasons for this including the high starch content and the fact that they have to be cooked which we have mentioned.

- Another problem is that of the grains, rice, the one normally chosen is about the worst, particularly if it is white rice. Even brown rice in large amounts will cause health problems for dogs.

I have seen large numbers of rice fed dogs over the years with cancer, pancreatic problems including diabetes, and arthritis. Each of these problems could be directly attributed to a lifetime spent eating a predominantly rice based diet. IF you must use grains, use less of them and use rolled oats instead or in addition.

- Replace those grains and legumes with many more green leafy vegetables, suitably prepared. That can include sprouted grains and legumes.

You mention bread. It is a highly processed product. Use it but not in large amounts.

Do add brewer's yeast as I have suggested. Apart from the B vitamins, it contains a glucose tolerance compound containing chromium. This compound helps stabilise blood sugar levels, particularly where a dog is being fed large quantities of cooked and therefore very digestible carbohydrates. By this means it helps prevent sugar diabetes.

- A major part of the problem of excessive grain is the low levels of zinc available to your dog.

This contributes to growth, reproductive, immune and skin problems plus pancreatic problems including Pancreatic Insufficiency, Pancreatitis, and sugar Diabetes.

The foods to add to a vegetarian diet to improve this situation are peas, carrots, cabbage and oatmeal. Alternatively, or in addition it would also be worthwhile to add a zinc supplement.

- Another major problem with most vegetarian diets based on grains is that they are low in essential fatty acids.

This lack will eventually produce a number of problems, the most obvious being skin problems. The solution is to add some vegetable oils to the diet. Soybean and corn oil would be the most logical because of their balance of the omega 3 and omega 6 groups of essential fatty acids.

In winter, particularly if your dog does not get much sun, add some cod liver oil for it's vitamin D content. The vitamin A which is also found in cod liver oil helps protect agains coughs and colds, so prevalent in the colder months of the year. It will also confer health in many other areas of your dog's life, including it's skin.

Some people also advocate a little apple cider vinegar daily. The unprocessed [expensive] stuff from your health food store. I do not know the scientific basis of the value of this. However a lot of dog owners swear by it as having immune stimulating effects. [That is what they mean even if they do not put it that way.. perhaps it is full of anti-oxidant type nutrients.]

- Grain based diets also tend to be low in the sulphur containing amino acids.

The two which worry me are Methionine and Taurine. Methionine is essential [amongst other things] for skin health, whilst Taurine is essential [amongst other things] for brain health.

A lack of taurine is a probable major cause of epilepsy. I have seen epilepsy disappear when a dog with the problem was taken off a dry dog food based on grain, and fed a balanced natural diet with a much higher Taurine content.

To ensure adequate sulphur in the diet, do add plenty of garlic and onions and chives etc. and also lots of green peppers. It is also not a bad idea to add some elemental sulphur. This is known as flowers of sulphur.

- Another problem is that this diet may be low in some minerals because of the lack of bones, dairy products and whole seafoods.

The one that worries me most is calcium. Another potential problem is a magnesium deficiency. The only really good plant source of calcium, apart from legumes, that I am aware of, is crushed sesame seeds or tahini. Magnesium is found in corn and also in fresh green leafy vegetables.

This may be a case where one of the complete mineral supplements will be of benefit. However, none of those have the same health promoting benefits of raw meaty bones.

Both kelp tablets and brewer's yeast help with any possible lack of trace minerals.

- Another problem feature of most vegetarian diets is that the vegetable or salad portion is poorly digested by the dog.

This happens when it is not prepared properly for a dog. That is, it is presented to the dog in very small quantities but in fairly large lumps.

Unless the salad vegetables are properly prepared, and there are sufficient of them, they are probably of very little value.

The only way to prepare vegetable material for a dog and that includes sprouted grains and sprouted legumes, corn kernels, carrots, celery , peas, beans, green leafy vegetables - whatever, is to turn them into a mush, much like the intestinal contents of a cow or a sheep.

One very good way to do that is to put them through a juicer and then remix the juice and the pulp and feed that to the dog. If that makes the mix too sloppy, drink some of the juice yourself!

- I know this diet will almost certainly be low in iodine because all Australian soils are low in iodine, which means the food they produce is also low in this important mineral.

Low iodine in your dog's diet does not allow your dog's thyroid to function properly, and if you are feeding lots of members of the cabbage family to your dog, it may also be causing the thyroid to be less active than it ought to be. This can interfere with growth reproduction, and the ability to have plenty of energy all day long. ADD SOME KELP DAILY.

CONCLUSION

Hope you and your veggie friends find this helpful. If you make the changes as I have suggested, those dogs will be a lot healthier. If you can see your way clear to adding some raw meaty bones [at least fifty percent of the diet would be great], and some eggs, you will indeed have a superbly healthy diet for your dogs.

Best wishes...........

- 22 -

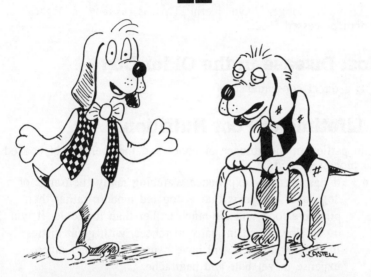

Feeding Your Dog For a Healthy Old Age

The modern dog like the modern dog's owner has fallen prey to the whole range of degenerative diseases. The number one killer of the older dog is cancer. This is followed by kidney disease and heart disease. Many older dogs suffer from arthritis, skin problems and bowel problems such as Pancreatitis. The very common disease in the modern human animal, Diabetes is also common in the older dog.

Many Older Dogs no Longer have Dental Problems.

They no longer have teeth! This is usually a legacy of modern processed foods.

Most Disease in the Older Dog -

Is a direct consequence of

A Lifetime of Poor Nutrition.

In particular, the absence of bones and the presence of cooked and processed foods.

- It has been my experience watching many thousands of dogs over the years that a dog fed modern rather than primitive food will die much earlier than it should. It will do so slowly and in many instances, with great distress. In the meantime it will have caused it's owner much expense in vet bills and heartache.

This chapter is about promoting the health of the older dog. It is about feeding the older dog to minimise disease, particularly the degenerative diseases. Diseases that in many people's minds are the inevitable consequences of growing old.

- Disease in old age is not inevitable. it is possible for your dog to live a longer, healthier life than many of you imagined possible. Health in your older dog depends on healthy eating. Principally the continuance of the raw meaty bone habit.

As an important background to the very simple principles involved in feeding the older dog, I will first discuss with you the ageing process.

Once you understand what ageing is, how it occurs, how it affects the health of your dog, and how it can be reduced to an absolute minimum, you will understand the importance of two types of foods.

- Firstly whole, raw, primitive foods, and -
- Secondly, mega-doses of certain nutrients.

Both of these have the ability to slow many aspects of the ageing process and thereby promote health.

AGEING - WHAT IS IT ?

Ageing does not mean getting older. Something can be very old but not aged. Ageing means deterioration. A slowing down process. Wearing out and loss of function. For your dog it means no body part functioning as well as it used to. Ultimately it ends in death, but on the way ageing produces a lot of ill health.

Most people regard ageing as inevitable. Something about which nothing can be done. Modern science is proving this to be untrue. We may not be able to maintain eternal youth, but there is a lot which can be done to slow the ageing process. When we do, there is an added bonus. Improved health. Our dogs are no exception.

Research is showing that sickness and ageing are very closely related. In fact they are almost the same thing. By slowing the ageing process, you are also promoting freedom from disease. By accelerating the ageing process, you can cause disease. This is such an important concept it would have been quite appropriate to discuss it in the section dealing with feeding puppies, particularly when you consider that ageing begins before your dog is born and continues for your dog's entire lifetime.

- Ageing consists of many different processes. Those processes fall into two broad groups. One group, programmed ageing we can do very little about. The other group of processes, the random ageing processes are the important ones so far as staying healthy is concerned.

Programmed Ageing

Ageing cannot be entirely prevented. You knew that already of course. All animals will eventually die. This is because each plant or animal on this earth, from the moment it begins life has a built in obsolesence. It has inherited a maximum lifespan. It has an ageing clock. This ageing clock is a bit like a time bomb.

It is a mechanism which eventually kills the organism. It is a series of maturation processes all creatures go through, which take them from youth to maturity, and finally to death.

A common example of programmed ageing that most of us are familiar with is the human female animal. She goes through childhood, followed by puberty followed by sexual maturity, followed by menopause, followed ultimately by death.

- This sort of ageing cannot be controlled by diet or drugs or by any other method except perhaps by breeding animals for longer life. It is the reason even the healthiest old animal or person will eventually die.

Over the period of an animal's lifetime, these ageing clocks first turn on and then gradually shut down various systems.

The final act of these biological ageing clocks is to cause an animal to self destruct or die. This will occur no matter how healthy the individual is at the time. However, it is rare for any human or animal to survive that long. This is because of the ravages of random ageing, a process I will talk about in just a moment.

Some simple examples of programmed ageing in the dog world can be seen at work if we consider the life spans of various breeds of dogs.

If your dog is a Saint Bernard, you will probably be aware that it has inherited a shorter span of life than a Poodle or a Kelpie.

- In general, smaller dogs live longer than large dogs. Humans live longer than dogs. These are examples of programmed ageing at work.

Because programmed ageing is a process we can do little or nothing about, I shall not discuss it further. It is the second process, random ageing, which is so vitally important. It is this process which is responsible for most of the health problems seen in dogs. The good news is that it is this process over which we can have a major degree of control.

Random Ageing - the Origins of Disease

Healthy young animals' bodies, like new cars, work really well. All the parts are new, and they are superbly protected by a healthy young immune system. So why don't they stay that way? Why do living things start to malfunction as they get older?

- The answer is, because they undergo random ageing.

Random ageing occurs when parts of the body break down and are repaired less than perfectly, leaving the body not able to function as well as it could previously.

Apart from inherited diseases and problems caused by trauma and poisoning, it is the process of random ageing, which is the chief cause of all diseases. A common example of this type of ageing is a breakdown in the immune system, resulting in problems such as infectious disease and cancer.

Random ageing can affect every organ system, in fact every cell in your dog's body. It results in progressive deterioration. It results in discomfort, disease and early death. It is common for animals to die earlier than they have to because of the effects of random ageing.

- Fortunately, random ageing, is a process over which it is possible to have very great control. It is possible for an animal or a person to undergo very little random ageing during it's lifetime.

Control of Random Ageing

Scientists studying ageing in a whole range of animals, including the dog and man are uncovering the relationship between food, disease and old age. They have found that many of the ageing or degenerative processes are hurried up or slowed down very much by what the subject eats. They have demonstrated that as animals and people, eat unsuitable food, or unsuitable amounts of food, they age or degenerate more rapidly, and as they do so, they become much more prone to disease.

- In other words, what you feed your dog, if you do it
  right, can actually slow the ageing process. If you can
  slow the ageing process, which is basically a process of
  deterioration and failure to repair, then you will also be
  on the right track to preventing disease.

In fact, depending on how much or how little time, effort and
money you are prepared to put into looking after your dog you
can choose your dog's rate of ageing and deterioration, and
therefore it's sickness level. It is totally your choice. You make
that choice by what you give and allow your dog to eat.

Speeding Up the Ageing Process

If you want your dog to age rapidly, have a short but miserable life, a life filled with ill health and unhappiness, then feed
it badly.

The simplest way to do that is to feed your dog commercial
dog food only. Another excellent method of accelerating the ageing process is to prepare the food yourself, making sure that it is
all cooked. Never feed your dog fresh uncooked food, and most
particularly do not feed it bones... ever.

There are plenty of other things you can do to ensure your
dog is not healthy, particularly as it gets older. You could feed it
an unbalanced diet such as all meat for example. One of the
most common ways people get their dog to break down is to
make sure their dog is over-fed. They encourage it to become
fat.

If your dog is already sick, then the simplest way to keep it
that way is to keep feeding it badly. Modern drugs will help to
alleviate many of the symptoms, and will often make it feel better. However, they will rarely slow the progression of the disease. They will not stop the ageing process. That requires a
change of diet.

- Of course nobody would deliberately harm their dog. The
  big problem is, so many people harm their dog without
  intending to by feeding it badly.

Slowing Down The ageing Process.

If you have read the first part of this book, you will know the sort of foods dogs have been designed to eat. You will know that a dog's basic diet should consist of raw meaty bones. You will know that most of it's food should be raw, and that it should consist of as wide a variety of foods as possible. You will know it is important that each meal is not complete and balanced with every nutrient it requires. You will know that balance must be achieved over many different meals. You will know that it should be kept slim and athletic.

- In other words, for maximum health, and a long life a dog should be kept on it's primitive diet for it's whole life.

If your dog is old with no teeth, you can and should continue to feed it bones ! How ?

That's simple - feed it minced up bones. E.g. minced up chicken wings. Use these as the basis of your old dog's diet.

DOES THAT MEAN FOR A DOG... NATURAL IS BEST ?

Many people feel that if only they can return their dog to nature, it will live a long happy and carefree life. These people believe that natural means best. That is not necessarily so.

Dogs in their natural state in the wild do not live much beyond five or six years of age.

- As far as nature is concerned, once a dog has reproduced itself, it is no longer necessary in the greater scheme of things. It no longer needs to stay alive. It can die. And it usually does !

In that sense, old age in animals is an unnatural event.

We artificially prolong our pet animals' lives. We do this in a number of ways, including preventative medicine programmes such as vaccination and worming, protecting them against natural enemies, providing shelter and warmth, providing food for which they don't have to hunt, and of course by medicating our dogs when they become ill.

- By doing all that for our dogs, we buy them extra time, well beyond the normal life expectancy. This is done, not by returning them to nature, but by creating a totally unnatural environment for them to live in.

We protect them from external attack. In other words, so far as external protection goes, unnatural is best for your dog because it prolongs your dog's life.

What about internal protection. Is unnatural best here ? The answer is yes and no. Let me explain.

- When people express the desire to return their dog to nature, they are wanting to feed it it's primitive diet. What they are actually talking about is feeding it to promote maximum health and immunity against disease. This is internal protection.

That is a great idea, and one which we have already discussed. By feeding your dog a primitive or natural diet you prolong it's life because you are using fuel, lubricants and spare parts which are specially designed for your dog by nature. You are maintaining it properly as you would a car with regular servicing, clean fuel, and genuine replacement parts. You are not using the inferior "el cheapo" products as produced by most dog food companies.

There is however, something unnatural which can be done for our dogs which will also help prolong their lives, and keep them free from disease. We can supply unnatural internal protection. Extra nutrients in a concentration possibly greater than is found in nature, and much much higher than is found in processed foods.

This is where science teams up with nature to help your dog.

- Not with processed foods which accelerate internal destruction, but with high doses of anti-oxidant nutrients.

This type of nutrient provides internal protection for your dog. Anti-oxidants slow down the processes of deterioration and destruction caused by random ageing.

Halting the Destruction Caused by Random Ageing

Random ageing is not one mechanism, but a series of mechanisms. In fact a series of processes within a living body, whereby it starts to break down, to wear out and no longer function properly.

It is these processes of ageing which raw whole foods combat so effectively. They do this for several reasons. One is because of the effects of food separation. Natural feeding or primitive feeding works on the basis that no meal contains every required nutrient. As discussed in Chapter 6, this method of feeding is much healthier for your dog. Most particularly it helps ensure kidney health, and it ensures that no vital nutrients become unavailable because of nutrient interactions.

The other, and perhaps more important way that primitive foods combat the ageing process is because they contain anti-degeneration nutrients known as anti-oxidants. These can include enzymes and other as yet unknown anti-ageing factors.

- Anti-oxidants are molecules which protect living bodies against the destructive attacks of molecules called free radicals.
- It is now widely accepted that damage by free radicals is a basic cause of random ageing.
- Destructive free radicals are produced both within the body and in the environment.

I do not wish to become bogged down in a discussion of the free radical theory of ageing. The important points you should be aware of are, that these dangerous molecules, these free radicals exist and they cause accelerated ageing, and to reduce ageing and help prevent disease, they must be destroyed.

Food is the principle source of supply of molecules which help scavenge and eliminate these free radicals. The free radical destroying molecules which are vital to a long and healthy life are called anti-oxidants.

- Many nutrients, and in particular vitamins, have a role as anti-oxidants. Nutrients that act as anti-oxidants include enzymes, sulphur containing amino acids, vitamins B1, B3, B5, B6, B12, vitamins A, C, E, and K, and also minerals such as zinc, selenium and chromium.

To be effective in their role of eliminating free radicals, some of these nutrients, the vitamins, need to be added to the diet in much larger amounts than has previously been thought necessary. The so called mega-doses, or fourth level of addition as discussed in Chapter 5. It is only when supplied at this level that they will successfully combat the ravages of ageing.

There are many as yet "unidentified" molecules present in whole raw foods which prevent ageing and fight disease. Similar molecules are the active ingredients in many of the medicinal herbs. Doubtless, most of these have anti-oxidant activity. This is a wide open field for research. New light on the role of these chemicals in retarding the ageing process and boosting the immune system is being shed every day.

- It is because many of these anti-ageing molecules are destroyed by heat, that cooked food, which of course includes processed food is so much less valuable in prolonging life and preventing disease than raw food.

YOUR DOG CAN DO BETTER

I want your dog to live a longer and healthier life than the majority of dogs today. I want your dog to live a long healthy life to the point where his or her body will have to be finally turned off as part of programmed ageing, because virtually no random damage has been caused.

You can do this for your dog. You can feed your dog in such a way that you will reduce the random damage to an absolute minimum. All you need do is feed your dog a primitive type of diet based on raw meaty bones as described in Chapter 18, and supplement that with appropriate doses of anti-ageing or anti-oxidant nutrients.

FEEDING YOUR OLDER DOG FOR LONG LIFE AND HEALTH

If you have not done so already, please read Chapter 18 which describes how to feed healthy adult dogs.

The "Do's"

- Do feed the sort of food that your dog evolved on.... that is, the food which your dog's body is genetically accustomed to eating. This means mostly whole raw foods. Primitive foods. Foods which have not been processed. That is, base your dog's diet on raw meaty bones.

- Do feed lots of fresh, leafy green vegetables suitably prepared. Apart from raw meaty bones, these should form the bulk of the rest of your older dog's diet. This is most important. You may add small amounts of protein foods such as minced meats, egg yolks, grated cheese and oils. You may also add brewer's yeast and kelp powder.

- Do feed small amounts of organ meats including liver, kidneys, brains and hearts on a regular basis. Note that they should not constitute more than about 10 % - 15 % of the diet.

- Do give your healthy older dog a regular fast of one to two days duration - every two weeks or so.

- Do watch your older dog's weight and general condition, and adjust size, frequency and content of food to maintain optimum weight and condition.

- Do feed only high quality protein foods, keeping poor quality proteins as found in commercial dog foods to a minimum. That means feeding plenty of eggs, cottage cheese, cheese, fresh mutton, fowl, beef, rabbit, fish, pork and most important of all... raw meaty bones !

- Do feed fat that has a high percentage of essential fatty acids. That means pig and chicken fat, vegetable oils such as sunflower, safflower, corn, canola, soyabean, linseed, sesame, grapeseed, olive etc., and fish oils.

- Do supplement fatty meals with vitamin E, selenium, and methionine. Your vet, or your health food store can supply all of these in tablet or capsule form. Alternatively, the selenium can be supplied in brewer's yeast and eggs, and the methionine can come from eggs.

- Do feed small amounts of offal once a week. E.g. liver and kidney.

- Do make sure you feed your dog a balanced regime of vitamins and anti-oxidant minerals. The vitamins should include the anti-oxidant vitamins fed at the third or fourth level.

The "Don'ts"

- In general, avoid all cooked and processed foods. These contribute heavily to a short and often very miserable life.

- Avoid food that contains excessive salt, protein, phosphorus and calcium.... which mostly means avoid processed foods.... avoid commercial dog foods. Do not feed those salty doggy treats.

- Do not allow your dog to become obese. In other words do not feed your dog too much food. Too much food means your dog becomes fat. Fat dogs have shorter lives than dogs of normal weight. This has much to do with free radical production by fat, and a lack of anti-oxidants in the diet.

- Do not feed your dog a lot of cereal grains or other starchy foods.

- Do not combine heavy starchy foods such as potatoes, grains, pasta etc with heavy protein foods such as meat, egg, cheese, fish.

In Summary

As you can see, it is absurdly simple. You are going to continue feeding your older healthy dog on a diet which is very similar to the one you fed your younger, healthy, non-reproducing, non-working dog.

That is, plenty of raw meaty bones fed by themselves, say about 50 % of the diet. Small amounts only of starchy foods, always fed without a concentrated protein source, but you can add veggies, and oil. Plenty of fresh, green leafy vegetables.

- As the dog gets older, the proportions of fresh, green leafy vegetables should be increased.
- With the older animal it is vitally important that meals which contain protein, contain only high quality protein as described.
- Protein and oil type foods can be added to the vegetable mush, and don't forget regular small amounts of offal foods, and the daily vitamin supplements.

Recommended Vitamin Supplements

The B Complex

This will be supplied by liver, green leafy vegetables, brewer's yeast etc. which you are already feeding. However, as discussed previously, you will do no harm by adding extra B's to your dog's diet.

See your chemist, vet, health food store, possibly your pet shop and purchase either a supplement designed specifically for dogs, or a human product.

A careful examination of the label of many vitamin supplements produced specifically for dogs, will reveal pretty low levels. Compare to a human product. In general, if using a human product, use half a child's dose for a small 10 kg dog, a child's dose for a 20 - 40 kg dog and an adult dose for a dog over 50 kg. These are a rough guide only. Because the B vitamins are so safe, so non toxic, even for a tiny 5 kg dog, the human adult dose would do no harm.

WARNING: do not give B vitamins on an empty stomach, they may cause vomiting.

Vitamin C

Any fresh fruit or green leafy vegetables fed to your older dog will supply some vitamin C. However, for a long and healthy life, do supply extra.

As a rough guide, use about 100 mg per kg. That means a 10 kg dog would receive about a gram of vitamin C per day, whereas a 50 kg dog would receive about five grams per day. This should be divided into at least two and preferably three doses.

For a healthy older dog, any of the different forms of vitamin C would do. However, if there is any question of health problems, please read the section on vitamin C in Chapter 5, which describes the different forms, including a few do's and don'ts.

Vitamins A and D

If you are feeding liver on a regular basis, it will most probably not be necessary to supply extra vitamin A. Also, if your dog does spend plenty of time in the sun, extra D may not be necessary.

However, many older dogs spend a lot of time indoors, particularly during the winter months, and they also become less able to efficiently use many nutrients including both A and D.

- WARNING: with these two vitamins, do be careful. If your dog has kidney problems, consult your vet before using either of them in supplementary form.

A and D are usually supplied together. If buying human grade vitamins, you will find capsules containing either 5 or 10 thousand international units of vitamin A together with an appropriate balancing amount of vitamin D.

As a rough guide, feed a 10 kg dog 2,500 to 5000 i.u. per day and a 50 kg dog between 10 000 and 20 000 i.u. per day. If you are also giving a substantial vitamin E supplement, these doses should be halved.

- It is quite a good idea to supply these two vitamins for a month, and then withold them for a month. The witholding period may be longer if your dog eats liver regularly.

Please read the section on vitamin A in Chapter 5. If unsure, please consult your vet. Both of you read it together !

Vitamin E

This is the anti-ageing vitamin par excellence ! With older dogs, it should be almost a criminal offence not to give it ! However, if your dog has any cardiovascular disease, the dose will have to begin small and be gradually increased. This is because if your dog has increased blood pressure, a large dose will temporarily make it go even higher.

However, by starting off at the lower dose rate, and gradually working up, there will be no problems. Do consult your vet.

The recommended dose rate is 10 to 20 mg [or i.u. - same thing] per kg per day. That is for a 25 kg dog, 250 to 500 mg per day. If in doubt about your dog's blood pressure, start at about one tenth that dose, and gradually work up to the desired dose over about a month. Get your vet to monitor this process.

Vitamin K

We now know that this has anti-aging properties, so it is worthwhile ensuring your older dog receives plenty one way or another.

Green leafy vegetables and liver will supply this vitamin. If giving extra, you may supply 1 - 10 mg of vitamin K per kg of dog per day. If using the synthetic form, do not go above this dose rate. [See Chapter 5.]

That's it for the moment. So until the next book arrives -

LET ME WISH YOU AND YOUR DOG[S] ---

---------------- **GOOD HEALTH** ----------------

BIBLIOGRAPHY

Airola Paavo, N.D., Ph.D. *"Hypoglycemia: a Better Approach."* Health Plus 1977.

Allcock James. Veterinary Surgeon. *"Pets in Particular."* Guild Publishing 1986.

Anderson, R.S. *"Nutrition of the Dog and Cat.* Pergamon Press 1980.

Anderson, R.S. *"Nutrition and Behaviour in Dogs and Cats."* Pergamon Press 1984.

Atrens, Dale M., Ph.d. *"Don't Diet "* A Bantam/Schwartz Book. 1988.

Australian Consumers' Asociation. *"How Safe is Our Food ?"* Random House Australia. 1991.

Ballentine, Rudolph, M.D. *"Diet & Nutrition - a Holistic Approach."* Published by The Himalayan International Institiute. 1978.

Banks, Josephine & Loeb, Paul. *"Nutrition and Your Dog."* Pocket Books 1984.

Belfield, Wendell O., D.V.M., & Zucker, Martin. *"How to have a Healthier Dog. The Benefits of Vitamins and Minerals for Your Dog's Life Cycles."* A Signet Book, 1981.

Berger, Stuart M., M.D. *"How to be Your Own Nutritionist."* A Bantam Schwartz Book. 1987.

Berger, Stuart M., M.D. *"What Your Doctor Didn't Learn in Medical School - and what You can Do About It."* Corgi and Bantam Books 1988.

Berger, Stuart M., M.D. *"Dr. Berger's Immune Power Diet."* A Bantam Schwartz Book. 1989.

Berman, Kathleen and Landesman, Bill. *"Caring For Your Older Dog."* David and Charles. 1985.

Best and Taylor's *"Physiological Basis of Medical Practice. Eleventh Edition."* Edited by John West, M.D., Ph.D. Williams and Wilkins 1985.

Blackshaw, Judith K., B.Sc., M.A.Ed., Phd. *"Notes on Some*

Topics of Applied Animal Behaviour." ISBN 0959258108. 1983.

Blogg, Rowan & Allan, Eric. *"Everydog. The Complete Book of Dog Care."* Methuen Australia, 1983.

Buist Robert PhD. *"Food Chemical Sensitivity."* Harper and Row 1986.

Carlson, Delbert G., D.V.M., and Giffin, James M., M.D. *"Dog Owner's Home Veterinary Handbook."* Howell Book House Inc. 1981.

Churchill, Jennie. B.V.Sc. *"Pet Sense."* Angus and Robertson 1990.

Clark, Linda. *"Know Your Nutrition."* Keats Publishing, Inc. 1984.

Cleave T.L., M.R.C.P. [London], *"The Saccharine Disease."* Keats Publishing Inc. 1975.

Cooper, Harry. B.V.Sc. *"Dr. Harry Cooper's Pet Care Guide."* Margaret Gee 1991.

Craighead George, Jean. *"How to Talk to Your Animals."* Hodder and Stoughton. 1985.

Crook William G., M.D. *"The Yeast Connection."* Professional Books 1983.

Davies, Dr. Stephen & Stewart, Dr. Alan. *"Nutritional Medicine."* Pan 1987.

De Bairacli Levy, Juliette. *"The Complete Herbal Book for the Dog."* Faber and Faber Limited. 1971. Dong Collin H., M.D. and Jane Banks. *"New Hope for the Arthritic."*

Grafton Books [Collins], 1976.

Drake, T.G.H. et al, *"The Biological Availability of Bone."* J. Nutr., 16:291.

Edney A.T.B., Editor, *"Dog and Cat Nutrition. A Handbook for Students, Veterinarians, Breeders and Owners."* Pergamon Press 1982.

Erdmann, Dr. Robert & Jones, Meiron. *"The Amino Revolution."* Century Paperbacks, 1987.

Faelton, Sharon, and the editors of Prevention Magazine. *"The Complete Book of Minerals for Health.* Rodale Press. 1981.

Fogle Bruce, Dr. *"Games Pets Play."* Methuen. 1986.

Goodman & Gilman. *"The Pharmacological Basis of Therapeutics. Fourth Edition"* Collier-Macmillan Limited 1970. Gracey, J.F., PhD., B.Agr., M.R.C.V.S., D.V.S.M., F.R.S.H. *"Thornton's Meat Hygiene."* Bailliere Tindall. 1981.

Grant, Doris & Joice, Jean. *"Food Combining for Health."* Thorsons, 1984.

Halvorsen, Brian. *"The Natural Dentist."* Century Arrow, 1986.

Hay, William Howard. M.D. *"Health via Food."* Edited and revised by Rasmus Alsaker. M.D. George G. Harrap & Co. Ltd. 1938.

Higgins Peter. B.V.Sc. *"New Idea Pet Care."* Southdown Press 1987.

Horne Ross. *"The Health Revolution. Fourth Edition."* Published by Happy Landings Pty Ltd. 1985.

Horne, Ross. *"Improving on Pritikin - You can do Better !"* Published by Happy Landings Pty Ltd. 1988.

Howell, Edward. Dr. *"Enzyme Nutrition. The Food Enzyme Concept."* Avery Publishing Group Inc. 1985.

Kenton, Leslie & Susannah. *"Raw Energy."* Doubleday. 1986.

Kirk. *"Current Veterinary Therapy X - Small Animal Practice."* W.B Saunders 1989.

Kronfeld D.S. Ph.D., D.Sc., M.R.C.V.S., A.C.V.I.M. Various papers in *"Proceedings No. 63 Nutrition."* Refresher Course for Veterinarians, 9 - 13 may 1983, The University of Sydney.

Lau, Benjamin. M.D.. Ph.D. *"Garlic For Health."* Lotus Light Publications 1988.

Lazarus, Pat. *"Keep Your Pet Healthy the Natural Way."* A Keats Pivot Health Book. 1983. Le Fanu, Dr., James. *"Eat Your Heart Out."* Macmillan London. 1987.

Lewis, Lon D., D.V.M., PH.D., Hand, Michael S., Seminar - *The Role of Dietary Management in Dog, cat and Horse Practice."* 28 November - 2 December 1988. Audio tapes held by The Post Graduate Committee in Veterinary Science of the University of Sydney. P.O. Box A561, Sydney South 2000. Ph.

[02] 264 2122.

Lewis Lon D., D.V.M., PH.D., et al, *"Small Animal Clinical Nutrition III."* Mark Morris Associates. 1987.

Mackarness, Richard. M.B. B.S., *"Eat Fat and Grow Slim."* The Harvill Press 1958.

Mackarness, Richard. M.B. B.S., D.P.M. *"Not all in the Mind."* Pan 1976.

MacLean & Graham, Drs. *Pediatric Nutrition in Clinical Practice."* The Addison-Wesley Clinical Practice Series.

Maynard and Loosli. *"Animal Nutrition. Fifth Edition."* Mcgraw-Hill, 1962.

McDowell, Lee Russell. *"Vitamins in Animal Nutrition. Comparative Aspects to Human Nutrition."* Academic Press Inc. 1989.

Mervyn, Leonard. B.Sc., Ph.D., C.Chem., F.R.S.C. *"The Dictionary of Vitamins."* Lothian Publishing Company Pty. Ltd. 1984.

Morris Desmond. *"Dogwatching."* Jonathan Cape. 1986.

Moser, Edward A. M.S., V.M.D. *"Dietary Fiber and it's Role in Veterinary Nutrition."* Publication by Hill's Pet Products. P.O Box 148 Topeka KS 66601, 913 354 8523.

Neville Peter. *"Do Dogs Need Shrinks ?"* Sidgwick and Jackson. 1991

McCarrison, Major General, Sir Robert, C.I.E., M.D., D.Sc., LL.D., F.R.C.P. *"Nutrition and National Health."* Faber and Faber 1936.

Mendelsohn, Robert S., M.D. *"Confessions of a Medical Heretic."* Warner Books. 1980.

Morrow, David A., D.V.M., Ph.D. *"Current Therapy in Theriogenology 2."* W.B. Saunders Company, 1986.

Nestel, Professor Paul J. Editor . *"Diet Health and Disease in Australia."* Harper and Row. 1987.

Pearson, Durk & Shaw, Sandy. *"Life Extension a Practical Scientific Approach."* Warner Books, 1982.

Pfeiffer, Dr, Carl C. *"Zinc and other Micronutrients."* A Pivot Original Health Book 1978.

Phillips David A. *"New Dimensions in Health. From Soil to Psyche."* Angus and Robertson Publishers. 1983.

Pitcairn Richard H. D.V.M., Ph.D., & Susan Hubbard Pitcairn. *"Dr. Pitcairn's Complete Guide to Natural Health for Dogs and Cats."* Rodale 1982.

Popper, Karl R. *"Conjectures and Refutations."* Routledge and Kegan Paul. 1962.

Rennie Neil. *"Working Dogs."* Shortland Publications Limited 1984.

Roach Peter. B.V.Sc., M.R.C.V.S., M.A.C.V.Sc. *"The Australian Women's Weekly Pet Care Book."* Published by Ita Buttrose. Sargent, Sarah. Rural writer for the Australian Financial Review. *"The Food makers."* Penguin Books. 1985.

Shaw, Susan. Vet Surgeon. *"Skin Allergy, Refresher Course for Veterinarians, Proceedings 139, 6, 7 & 8 July 1990.* Post Graduate Committee in Veterinary Science University of Sydney.

Sheffey, Professor Ben E. et al, *"Nutrition Seminar, Dogs - Cats - Greyhounds - Proceedings from."* The Post Graduate Committee in Veterinary Science, University of Sydney, 1974.

Smith, Lendon. M.D. *"Feed Yourself Right."* Doubleday. 1984.

Soulsby, E, J, L. M.A., Ph.D., M.R.C.V.S., D.V.S.M. *"Helminths, Arthropods, & Protozoa of Domesticated Animals."* Bailliere, Tindall and Cassell. 1971.

Stanton, Rosemary. *"Rosemary Stanton's Complete Book of Food and Nutrition."* Simon & Schuster, 1989.

Stedmans Medical Dictionary. 22nd Edition. Williams and Wilkins, 1972.

Stryker, Lubert. *"Biochemistry. Second Edition."* Freeman, 1981.

Swenson, Melvin J. D.V.M., M.S., Ph.D. Editor. *"Duke's Physiology of Domestic Animals. Eighth Edition."* Cornell University Press. 1970.

Taylor Renee. *"Hunza health Secrets for Long Life and Happiness."* Keats Publishing Inc. 1964.

Thompson, R., C., Andrew, B.Sc., Ph.D., D.I.C. *"Echinococcosis / Hydatidosis [in Australia]."* Proceedings 194. Zoonoses, Australian Veterinarians in Public Health. Published by Post Graduate Committee in Veterinary Science, University of Sydney.

Trum Hunter, Beatrice. *"Additives Book."* Keats Publishing 1980.

Udall, Robert H., & McCay, Clive M., *"The Feed Value of Fresh Bone"*

J. Nutr. V. 49, P. 197 1953.

Wahlqvist, Professor Mark, et al. *"Use and Abuse of Vitamins."* Sun Books 1987.

Watson, Lyall. Dr. *"Omnivore."* Corgi Books. 1973.

PERIODICALS

Australasian Health and Healing. Editor Maurice Finkel B.Sc.. MSc., MEd., Ed.D., N.D. Publisher:Trim Keg Pty. Ltd. Various editions and articles.

Australian Wellbeing. Publisher and Editor Barbara McGregor. Various editions and articles.

International Clinical Nutrition Review. Editor Robert A Buist Ph.D. Integrated Therapies Pty Ltd. Various Editions and Articles.

Waltham International Focus. Various issues.

OTHERS

Veterinary Pharmaceuticals and Biologicals. Fourth ed. 1985/ 1986. Editor Dr. Carl E. Aronson. Published by Veterinary Medicine Publishing Company.

Nutrition Almanac. John D. Kirschman. Mcgraw Hill Book Company. 1979.

Recommended Dietary Intakes for use in Australia. National Health and Medical Research Council. Australian Government Publishing Service Canberra. 1991.

Nutritional Values of Australian Foods. National Food Authority. Australian Government Publishing Service Canberra. 1991.

The Nutrient Composition of Australian Meats and Poultry. Food Technology in Australia 39: 181 - 240; 1987.